IN THE BLOOD

IN THE BLOOD

How Two Outsiders Solved a
Centuries-Old Medical Mystery and
Took On the US Army

CHARLES BARBER

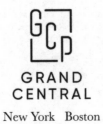

GRAND
CENTRAL
New York Boston

Grand Central Publishing
Hachette Book Group
1290 Avenue of the Americas, New York, NY 10104
grandcentralpublishing.com
twitter.com/grandcentralpub

First Edition: May 2023

Grand Central Publishing is a division of Hachette Book Group, Inc. The Grand Central Publishing name and logo is a trademark of Hachette Book Group, Inc.

The publisher is not responsible for websites (or their content) that are not owned by the publisher.

The Hachette Speakers Bureau provides a wide range of authors for speaking events. To find out more, go to hachettespeakersbureau.com or email HachetteSpeakers@hbgusa.com.

Grand Central Publishing books may be purchased in bulk for business, educational, or promotional use. For information, please contact your local bookseller or the Hachette Book Group Special Markets Department at special.markets@hbgusa.com.

Library of Congress Cataloging-in-Publication Data
Names: Barber, Charles, author.
Title: In the blood : how two outsiders solved a centuries-old medical mystery and took on the US Army / Charles Barber.
Other titles: How two outsiders solved a centuries-old medical mystery and took on the US Army
Description: First edition. | New York : Grand Central Publishing, 2023. | Includes index.
Identifiers: LCCN 2022057893 | ISBN 9781538709863 (hardcover) | ISBN 9781538709887 (ebook)
Subjects: LCSH: Medicine, Military—United States—History—20th century. | Hemorrhage—Treatment—United States—History—20th century. | Surgical dressings—History—20th century. | Wound treatment equipment industry—History—20th century.
Classification: LCC UH223 .B37 2023 | DDC 616.9/8023—dc23/eng/20221209
LC record available at https://lccn.loc.gov/2022057893

ISBN: 9781538709863 (hardcover), 9781538709887 (ebook)

Printed in the United States of America

LSC-C

Printing 1, 2023

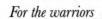

For the warriors

No army can withstand the strength of an idea whose time has come.
—Victor Hugo, "The History of a Crime," 1877

Contents

PRELUDE: *Mogadishu, 1993*   *xi*

   PART ONE: The Man Who Saw the Caverns

      Chapter One: The Simplest Idea   3

      Chapter Two: All Bleeding Stops Eventually   13

      Chapter Three: The Salesman with Nothing to Sell   28

   PART TWO: The Wars

      Chapter Four: The Rower   51

      Chapter Five: The Wound-Dresser   72

      Chapter Six: Already Dead   89

      Chapter Seven: "You burn people!"   114

      Chapter Eight: The Danger of Using a Sledgehammer to Crack a Nut   142

      Chapter Nine: Emotional Bankruptcy   171

   PART THREE: The Finish Line

      Chapter Ten: *United States v. Novo Nordisk*   185

      Chapter Eleven: The Army's Greatest Invention   198

POSTSCRIPT: *The Left Side of the Menu*   218

Prelude

Mogadishu, 1993

He who wishes to be a surgeon should go to war.
                                    —Hippocrates (460–370 BC)

AT 1:00 P.M. ON October 3, 1993, in the blinding white sunlight of an East African afternoon, a hundred Army Rangers rappelled down ropes from nineteen Black Hawk helicopters onto the dusty streets of the city of Mogadishu, in Somalia. Simultaneously, sixty soldiers drove into the city in a convoy of Humvees. The two groups were planning to converge within a two-block radius of a white stucco house in the center of Mogadishu. American and North American Treaty Organization (NATO) intelligence officials had ascertained that this house was the headquarters of General Mohamed Aidid. Their mission was to apprehend General Aidid, a warlord who had been starving hundreds of thousands of his fellow Somalis to death in a perverse display of power. A protracted conflict between Aidid and his rivals, which often involved indiscriminate shooting and bombing, had killed tens of thousands more.

Much of the populace lived in stick huts, and up to five thousand homeless boys roamed the streets. The city's white or pink stucco buildings were riddled with bullet holes, and many of the cars scattered along the streets amounted to little more than rusting carcasses. The only things that were undeniably beautiful about Mogadishu were its long stretches of beach and the iridescent, teal-colored waters of the Indian Ocean.

The army's plan, hatched in concert with NATO advisers, was to surround Aidid's headquarters, arrest him and his closest lieutenants, and once and for all rid the country of his rule. As the American soldiers descended and approached the white house, the warlord's men—more a street gang than an actual militia—fired at them with mainly third-rate rifles, the bullets pinging harmlessly off the impenetrable armor of the helicopters and Humvees. After all, Aidid's men—many of whom were teenagers—were equipped with mainly rifles and grenades, had little to no training, and were half-starving themselves. The first Rangers to hit the ground sprinted in short bursts toward Aidid's headquarters, pausing for cover in broken-down, sagging houses and alleyways. They drew fire, but the shots directed at them were erratic.

In the beginning, everything went according to plan. The military strategists—both Americans and advisers from NATO forces—believed that the mission would be accomplished within ninety minutes. The strategists reasoned that Aidid's supporters were amateurish, and the Americans, after all, had overwhelmingly superior firepower. The Black Hawks—each more than twenty yards long and weighing ten tons—were the most sophisticated helicopters ever built. The conflict was expected to be little more than a quick "snatch-and-grab" operation.

But early on, there was a bad omen. A soldier rappelling from one of the helicopters lost his grip and fell ninety feet to the ground. He survived, but his back was badly broken. Minutes later, the near-million-to-one shot happened. As one of the Black Hawks hovered just above the city, something hit its tail. At first not even the crewmen were aware that anything significant had occurred. But then the helicopter groaned and chortled—pausing momentarily in the air, as if affronted—and started to spin. The downward spiral began slowly at first but then gained ever greater force and velocity. The machine fell to the earth in a matter of seconds with a kind of shocking violence. In its final gyration, the helicopter clipped off the entire top half of a house and then rolled onto its side like a dying animal. It settled in the road, steam and fire rising from the wreckage. The two pilots were killed instantly. Remarkably, the six other crew members survived; four of them exited from the side door of the helicopter and attempted to secure the immediate area. They were met with a barrage of gunfire. One of the crew members killed perhaps ten Somalis before he himself was slain with four shots to the pelvis and abdomen. Miraculously, the people inside the house cleaved by the helicopter had survived.

The Black Hawk had been hit by an RPG—a rocket-propelled grenade. Before the conflict, the military strategists had considered this essentially a physical impossibility. In their faulty estimation, RPGs were effective only in ground warfare and had a meager range of three hundred yards. Furthermore, shooting one into the sky, as one of Aidid's men had had the temerity to do, was considered suicidal. The backblast was powerful enough to kill a man, and the very act of firing would instantly identify the location of the shooter to the helicopter marksmen. One could reasonably expect to be mowed down within seconds of launching the rocket.

Leave no man behind is perhaps the fundamental maxim drilled into an infantry soldier, and this is particularly true for a force as elite as the Rangers. With the helicopter down, the conflict pivoted immediately from a search-and-destroy operation to apprehend Aidid to a rescue mission to save the wounded and stranded soldiers. The Rangers in the Humvees were redirected away from

Aidid's hideout and toward their brethren pinned down around the fallen helicopter. In a matter of seconds, the battle transformed into an old-fashioned mano a mano brawl. And here the Americans' vaunted technology was of far less use. Clearly this had been the Somalis' plan all along—to quite literally bring the Americans down to earth. On the streets were the smells of rotten fruit, raw sewage, and gunpowder, and now the whoosh of overhead RPGs and screams of "Medic!" and "I'm hit!" Aidid's men believed that the Americans' apparent strengths—their glorious helicopters and armor, their goggles and infrared sensors, which the Africans believed made them look inhuman—also signaled their weakness. All that technology and protective gear, to the Somalis, meant that Americans were afraid to die. Now emboldened, Aidid's ragtag militia charged out onto the streets, and the Americans were soon encountering gunfire from rooftops, doorways, and alleys in every direction.

Then the unthinkable happened again. A second Black Hawk was hit by an RPG and crashed a mile from where the first helicopter had fallen. Three crew members were killed, either on impact or in the vicious fighting that immediately ensued, and a fourth was eventually captured. The Americans now had to attempt two simultaneous rescue operations. The anticipated hour-long engagement turned into twenty-seven hours of urban combat, the longest sustained conflict in which the American military had been engaged since Vietnam.

Some hours later, in the Forty-Sixth Combat Support Hospital, a temporary hospital made up of interconnected air-conditioned tents a few kilometers from the battle on the streets of Mogadishu, surgeon and US Army major John Holcomb did not know when the causalities were going to arrive. Holcomb, who had been given short notice that he was being deployed to Somalia, had spent his brief time there playing volleyball and having fun with members of his unit while also conducting medical trainings and preparing the combat hospital for action. Earlier that morning, Holcomb had operated on a little Somali girl whose face had been run over by a Humvee. A few days earlier, an Army Ranger, defying warnings, had splashed around in the water for an hour only to have his legs bitten off by a shark. John Holcomb had performed the initial operation on the solider, who was then airlifted to the army's hospital in Germany, accompanied by one of the doctors assigned to the Forty-Sixth Combat Hospital. The soldier died in Germany, and Holcomb's already thin team of surgeons was reduced from four doctors to three. Holcomb, as he waited in the Forty-Sixth Combat Support Hospital, knew that casualties of war were coming, but he did not know how many, nor when. In the end, he was given only ten seconds' notice that casualties were inbound.

Despite his relative youth—he was in his midthirties—Major Holcomb had been preparing for a moment like this all his life. He was by nature a confident man, and he had been well trained for whatever lay ahead of him. Holcomb seemed to be imbued with a supreme sense of certainty about things, an inveterate optimism, and the belief that the world, even while he waited on the edge of a battlefield, was something that one could manage and control. He once said there were no true car accidents. If people drove safely, were sober, and wore seat belts, there would essentially be no accidents. "When you look at it that way, 'accidents' are really predictable."

Holcomb grew up in the 1960s and 1970s in Fort Smith, Arkansas—known chiefly for having the lowest cost of living in the United States and for being the manufacturing and processing centers for the Planters peanut and Mars companies. He was able to go to medical school only because the military paid for it. He chose the army because his father had been an army officer for twenty-three years. After receiving his medical degree from the University of Arkansas in 1985, he completed his residency in general surgery at an army medical center and then became a staff surgeon at Fort Bragg in North Carolina and finally director of a US Army clinic in Turkey. In 1989 he was a surgeon in a special operations forces operation in Panama. He was specially trained for raids and assault missions.

Surely adding to Holcomb's sense of confidence was how relatively well equipped the Forty-Sixth Combat Support Hospital was, even if it was all in tents. Holcomb would later call it "a very capable hospital." The facility had three operating rooms, twelve intensive care unit beds, and thirty general ward beds. It had basic lab, X-ray, and CT scan capabilities. But then again, Holcomb was one of only three doctors on staff. Although they were not expected, if many casualties were to arrive, he and his small team were going to be in trouble.

And indeed, over the next thirty-six hours, Major John Holcomb and the two other doctors were overwhelmed by casualties. The wounded and the dying arrived in two waves, one at 5:30 p.m. on October 3 and the second at 6:00 a.m. on October 4. Out of the two hundred combatants in the conflict, 112 were injured and seventy were hospitalized. Holcomb and his colleagues performed thirty-four operations over a day and a half. The first three or four patients Holcomb operated on died. One soldier, whose leg had been blown off at the hip by a grenade, which severed his iliac artery, perished despite being given forty-six pints of blood. At one point a fellow surgeon looked in on Holcomb only to find him elbow deep in a young soldier's abdomen. At another point the power went out, and Holcomb operated by flashlight. Of one casualty Holcomb said more than a decade later, "He bled to death in my hands. It was horrible." Holcomb would refer to the entire blood-soaked episode as "the defining experience of my life."

As they attempted to save the lives of soldiers, the surgeons used gauze and pressure and ligatures—the same tools and techniques to stop traumatic bleeding that had been used since the Civil War. It was an excruciating, harrowing experience. "To have those soldiers bleed to death—and not be able to stop that bleeding—is so frustrating," Holcomb would say later. All told, eighteen Rangers died in the Battle of Mogadishu, and most likely thousands of Somalis—although the exact number of Somali casualties is unknown. But in the end, John Holcomb performed valiantly, even heroically: he did everything that a battlefield surgeon could be expected to do, and more.

———————

In the days and months and years after the conflict, the Battle of Mogadishu was widely considered a military and strategic disaster. The American public was shocked and repulsed by the images of the street fighting that were broadcast on television the next day. The day after the battle, Canadian photojournalist Paul Watson took a photograph of the half-naked corpse of an American soldier—a victim of the second Black Hawk crash—with his genitals exposed as he was dragged through the streets by a cheering crowd. The photograph would go on to win the Pulitzer Prize. The wretchedness and tawdriness of the image was simply too much for the American public to stomach. As Mark Bowden, the author who chronicled the battle in the best-selling book *Black Hawk Down: A Story of Modern War*, later wrote, the events in Mogadishu took place during a high-water mark of American military prestige, just two years after the Persian Gulf War. Victory in that conflict had been attained so quickly, and had incurred so few casualties, that most Americans had come to believe that their military was virtually unassailable. It seemed almost inconceivable that an elite American force could be overrun by what appeared on television to be a barely clothed and starving mob, or that the most advanced military technologies in the world could be felled by a simple grenade. The American commander of the operation quickly resigned in disgrace.

The hangover from Mogadishu was long lasting. American public opinion swiftly turned against interventionalist policies, and President Bill Clinton ordered all American soldiers to withdraw from Somalia by early 1994. Other Western nations followed suit. UN peacekeepers left the country in 1995, bringing to a close an unsuccessful mission that had cost billions of dollars and still left Somalia without a functional government. America showed no willingness to intervene in the genocide in Rwanda one year later, and in 1996, Osama bin Laden cited Watson's photograph as proof that the US was unable to tolerate the brutality of war. When "one American was dragged in the streets of Mogadishu," he said, "you left. The extent of your impotence and weaknesses became very clear."

In 2000, seven years after Mogadishu, John Holcomb, now director of trauma research for the army, delivered what amounted to a kind of postmortem analysis of the battle. Immediately after Mogadishu, he considered leaving the army and even had a contract to enter private practice in New Mexico, but he changed his mind at the last minute. He reflected later, "I came back from [Mogadishu], and it turned my career a hundred and eighty degrees. . . . We had a lot of soldiers bleed to death. . . . I came back and said, 'We need to figure out better ways to stop bleeding.'" He had not previously been oriented toward the idea of becoming a research scientist, but he'd spent the years since 1993 rising in the ranks of army medical research, and he'd worked relentlessly to develop a bioengineered bandage that would stem volume bleeding.

On March 23, 2000, he spoke in Santa Monica, California, at a conference organized by the RAND Corporation, a public policy think tank. The event was also sponsored by the US Army Training and Doctrine Command, the Marine Corps Warfighting Laboratory, and the Office of the Secretary of Defense.

In his remarks Holcomb spoke of the urgency of making advances in hemorrhage control. "Unfortunately, we are currently surrounding our soldiers with incredible technology, and yet the way we do hemorrhage control in the year 2000 is exactly the same way that it was done in the Trojan War, World War I, and World War II. We use the same gauze battle dressing that we have for decades. In the operating room we use gauze dressings, silk ties, and ligatures." He said that he and his colleagues hoped to field their bioengineered bandage in the next couple of years. Other countries, he pointed out, were already implementing investigational medical technologies such as advanced dressings, drugs that controlled bleeding, and blood substitutes, but the American military was unable to do so because of Food and Drug Administration restrictions. He argued that regulatory bodies—such as the FDA and the Joint Commission on Accreditation of Healthcare Organizations (JCAHO), which accredits hospitals—should not have jurisdiction in the field. In fact, he said, "The FDA and JCAHO do not exist in the field." Those entities, he said, did not understand the unique nature and urgency of combat medicine and were holding the military back on the battlefield by not allowing treatments that involved certain levels of risk. He criticized a US Department of Defense rule that required trauma patients to give individual consent, which stifled research and "essentially prohibited" the Pentagon from funding research in trauma. "We can't get better if we can't try new ways," he said. He called for writers of military medical doctrines to advance "rapid" and "relevant" techniques, even if those techniques were "unproved [sic] but [made] sense."

At the conclusion of his speech, Holcomb presented a slide that outlined in clear and direct language his definition of the ideal combat doctor, nurse, or medic. He quoted the *Emergency Ward Surgery* reference book that stated the ideal providers of trauma medicine in the combat environment were "young people who must have good hands, a stout heart, and not too much philosophy. They are called upon for decisions rather than discussion, for action rather than knowledge of what the latest writers think should be done."

Two years after his remarks, America would turn to war again, in Afghanistan and Iraq, and John Holcomb would soon become the director of the entirety of army trauma medicine. In that capacity he would hold absolutely true to every word of his own cited definition of the ideal combat doctor. Under his medical command, as hundreds of thousands of American soldiers fought in the war on terror, he indeed valued action over discussion, often ignored the latest medical literature, and willingly accepted risky techniques—even if they were "unproved"—to save lives. It appeared that his experiences at the Battle of Mogadishu had irrevocably altered him, and that he would do anything possible not to have soldiers bleed to death in his hands ever again.

PART ONE

THE MAN WHO SAW THE CAVERNS

Talent hits a target no one else can hit. Genius
hits a target no one else can see.
                                    —Arthur Schopenhauer

CHAPTER ONE

The Simplest Idea

IN THE FALL of 1983, Frank Hursey was a very happy man. At forty, he had been contentedly married to his wife, Nancy, a nurse, for the last fifteen years; he had thriving children, two girls and a boy; and he lived in a modest but comfortable house in the leafy and pleasant suburb of West Hartford, Connecticut. Frank was an untroubled person by nature. A lean man of medium height, with thick and just slightly graying brown hair and a relatively unlined face, Frank was the kind of person—mild mannered and unintimidating—that strangers approached on the street to ask for directions.

A mechanical engineer by training, he had been the first in his family to go to college. Over a period of ten years, he went to night school while working full-time during the day to earn a bachelor's degree from the University of Hartford. He then got a master's degree in business administration from Rensselaer Polytechnic Institute. This degree, he would joke, took him only six years to finish. When Frank was a teenager, his mother, a strong-willed woman and a devout Catholic, had suggested that her son read Norman Vincent Peale's self-help book *The Power of Positive Thinking*, which counseled its readers to immediately replace negative thoughts with more placid and hopeful ones. Over the course of his life, Frank had succeeded at following that advice to a rather remarkable degree. Now, on the cusp of middle age, his life was full and busy, with Boy Scout pack meetings and school plays, Mass on Sundays, dinners with Nancy and their small circle of friends, but most of all his work. With rare exceptions, he conducted his life and his affairs in an unruffled manner and with an optimistic spirit.

Frank had grown up poor in Dillon, South Carolina, the small and largely indigent town in the pinewoods and swamplands of the central part of the state. The main industry—really the sole industry—was timber and pulp and paper processing. His father, who had suffered from the effects of polio since childhood, died in his early fifties, most likely from being poisoned by the lead he used daily in his work as a Linotype operator at a newspaper printing plant. When Frank was sixteen, he surprised his father one day at work. It was the end of the shift, and Frank watched as his father punched out on the time clock. Frank never forgot the look of shame that cloaked his father's face in that moment. Frank made a promise to himself that one day he would have a career in which he did not have to work on anybody else's schedule. Frank went on to the University of South Carolina on a full scholarship, but was asked to leave during his freshman year because he couldn't concentrate on his coursework. He was too distracted and upset by his father's decline, and indeed, his father died not long after Frank left college. Frank's father spent his final weeks in a hospital two blocks from the family's home. In those last days, when Frank stood on the sidewalk outside the hospital, he could hear his father screaming in pain from his sickbed inside. After the death, the family—Frank, his mother, and his two sisters, one of whom had Down syndrome—moved to Connecticut, where they were taken in by an uncle who worked as a union organizer.

Frank immediately took to Connecticut: he liked the cooler climate, the defined seasons, the greater tolerance for his family's Catholic religion, and the fact that there were job opportunities in industry and technology. He met Nancy at a party and married her six months later. He was only twenty-one. Soon only a tinge of his South Carolina accent remained. Frank immediately got a job as an engineer's assistant at the huge defense contractor Pratt & Whitney, and, with his employer paying the tuition, enrolled at the University of Hartford. After a decade at Pratt, he became an engineer in the respiratory department at Hartford Hospital. Now, at the age of forty, he was about to set up his own company, which would manufacture machines that produced oxygen and nitrogen. This would be his third go-around at starting his own business: he had already failed at two previous attempts. One of the companies simply couldn't pay its bills, and at the second, Frank discovered that his business partner failed to pay taxes and then disappeared. The IRS investigators found Frank and threatened to repossess his house.

These experiences of course were deeply frustrating, but really what Frank most cared about was how things in the physical world worked and how to make them work better. He would walk by a streetlight and wonder about the wattage of the bulb, or examine a cappuccino maker and speculate on the pressure at which the gauge best operated. These types of things were deeply fascinating, and also amusing and pleasurable, to him. All things being equal, left to his own devices, he primarily thought of the world as a mechanical and logical place, governed by liquids and gases and vacuums and pressures. When he was simply driving around town or taking a walk or brushing his teeth, he enjoyed thinking about how these physical elements worked together, or against each other, like some gigantic, beautiful, and slightly mysterious apparatus.

But as a result, when he tried to explain the machines he built to customers, he wouldn't say what the machines could actually do for them—how they could supply nitrogen to a storage area to preserve otherwise perishable food products or create pure oxygen to ignite a flame capable of cutting metal. Instead, mostly he talked about the obscure science behind them, such as pressure swing technology, which separated gases in air by putting them under pressure and forcing them into a pervious material, often a mineral called zeolite, that absorbed some gases more readily than others. Frank used zeolite frequently in his machines; he found that oxygen passed through the mineral much more easily than nitrogen, making the resulting gas oxygen-enriched.

Frank was fascinated by zeolite, which looked like kitty litter and was just an inexpensive and inert mineral, strip-mined by Union Carbide in the American South. When he first encountered the rock, he was a student at the University of Hartford, and he went to the library to read scientific articles on the mineral so he could learn everything about it. Frank learned that zeolite had been used for millennia as a building material—large parts of ancient Rome and Naples were made of the rock—and that starting in the twentieth century, it had had a wide array of industrial uses: in the absorption of radiation in nuclear waste (it was employed successfully at Chernobyl); in the removal of ammonia from drinking water; as a deodorizer in pet litter, athletic footwear, and ashtrays; and as an ammonia filter in dialysis units. As Frank considered these myriad uses, he realized that they all had one thing in common: zeolite elegantly absorbed things, separating the elements of a given chemical. Whether it was applied to radiation, ammonia, molecules that created unpleasant smells, or nitrogen in air, the industrialists who used zeolite understood that the mineral captured the offending element. It was the perfect natural sieve. Poring over the literature, Frank studied the crystalline structure of the mineral and learned that about 50 percent of it was comprised of empty spaces—little caverns or, as Frank thought of them, "void spaces." In the electron microscope images of zeolite crystals that he found, Frank saw what zeolite looked like inside: a series of end-lessly repeating honeycomb patterns. The total surface area of the spaces or caverns within these honeycombs was truly astonishing, mind-boggling even. A heaping tablespoon of ground-up zeolite had the surface area of a football field.

Frank now understood that it was the caverns in zeolite's molec-ular structure that captured things. He now saw that some atoms and molecules were small enough to be trapped in the honey-combs. Had Frank worked with other scientists, he would have discussed his insights with them, but he was working entirely on his own. Frank wasn't sure if anyone else in the world could see the caverns of zeolite the way that he did, nor did he particularly care. Frank just knew that there was something magical about them, and he wondered if those caverns might be capable of doing even greater things.

In the fall of 1983, as he stood in his basement in the West Hartford house, with Nancy in the living room upstairs, Frank had an idea—a theory, really—that, if correct, might change his precarious financial situation. He was about to conduct an experi-ment. Frank's concept—the culmination of something he'd been turning over in his mind for years—was that the caverns in zeolite could capture elements in blood. Frank didn't know too much about blood, but he knew that it was mainly composed of water and that the remainder was made up of platelets and proteins, which were what caused it to clot. His idea was that the water molecules, which were small and simple, would get caught in the honeycombs, while the platelets and clotting proteins, much more complex and larger molecules, would be too big to be confined. The zeolite would act like a sponge, mopping up the water in blood, and what remained would be supersaturated with the elements that actually formed clots, thereby dramatically speeding up the clotting process. It was all a matter of simple arithmetic, really: addition by subtraction. To Frank, that was nothing but pure logic. And if he was correct—if zeolite led to blood being able to clot much more quickly—then maybe he could develop a product to help with shaving cuts, and this would make him rich. Or, if not that, at least allow him to successfully establish his own company.

It was a sunny Saturday morning in October, the time of year when, if it's not raining, Connecticut shimmers with a kind of golden sunlight that illuminates everything. He had bought a mouse at a pet store that morning. In his basement workshop, he was preparing to cut the mouse superficially with a razor. Upstairs, Nancy was shouting to him, "Frank, what are you doing with that poor mouse?" Frank had told her that he didn't want to hurt the creature—he had grown up hunting all kinds of animals in South Carolina, which was what everybody did in Dillon, but had since happily given it up—but if his theory was correct, the mouse was going to be OK. And, he told Nancy, there was a larger purpose in mind. Nancy severely doubted that. She was used to Frank and his big ideas. She thought all of them were interesting but had learned that few of them ever really led anywhere. At one point, in order to help his children focus on their homework, Frank had built a meter and attached it to the television set. If not fed with quarters, which the children didn't have, the meter would shut the TV off after half an hour. The contraption worked, but after a while everyone else in the family got annoyed with it and mad at Frank for inventing it in the first place.

Now, alone in the basement, Frank made a small incision in the mouse's belly, which produced a burst of blood, and then he inserted into the tiny wound a pinch of zeolite. He felt a surge of nervous anticipation as he waited to find out what would happen next. He immediately saw the blood thickening in the mouse's wound. Could this really be happening, or was it a trick of the mind? He watched in amazement as, a few seconds later, the blood moved even more slowly, becoming almost like Jell-O in its consistency. Then it stopped moving *entirely*, as if defying gravity. Just as he expected, the water had been captured in the caverns. The mouse had immediately developed a clot and had stopped bleeding entirely within twenty seconds or so. It easily survived, and Frank released it into his yard later that day.

After the experiment, Frank ran up the stairs to tell Nancy the results. She was far more interested in hearing that the mouse had lived. But with the success of his experiment, Frank began using zeolite on his cheek when he cut himself shaving. The blood dried up immediately. Some weeks later, Frank called up an old colleague, a surgeon at Hartford Hospital, and together they received permission to test zeolite on pigs after hours. A major research institution, the hospital already had animal testing protocols in place. The zeolite stopped the pigs' bleeding every time, in a matter of seconds. It was miraculous. There was now no doubt that zeolite was extraordinary at clotting blood, but Frank did observe one potential problem: occasionally he would notice heat around the tissue surrounding the wound after the zeolite was applied. He postulated that the absorption of the water molecules into the zeolite was so intense that it agitated them, which created friction, which in turn generated heat. He measured the temperatures, which could rise to 150 degrees Fahrenheit, hot enough at times to cause a mild burn.

On April 24, 1984, Frank submitted an application to the US Patent and Trademark Office, claiming that zeolite worked as a molecular sieve to stop bleeding in warm-blooded animals. The patent application was eccentrically written by Frank's attorney, and the submission contained spelling mistakes and run-on sentences. It took five years, but on April 18, 1989, Frank received a return letter stating that his patent had been accepted. Frank then wrote ten letters to drug, medical device, and personal care companies ranging from Pfizer and Eli Lilly to Schick and Gillette, telling them that he might have something that could be used to help with shaving accidents, or maybe other small cuts. He waited with great anticipation for their enthusiastic responses.

But only one of the companies bothered to send a reply— a withering sneer of a rejection letter from Johnson & Johnson. It appeared that even if he had a patent, no one was interested in the apparently grandiose claims of an obscure mechanical engineer in Connecticut. For a short time, Frank was annoyed and disappointed, even hurt, but he was not one to hold grudges.

Besides, two years later, in that third attempt at having his own company, he had succeeded, if only barely. The company was called On-Site Gas Systems. Frank rented a grimy workshop with manufacturing space in a corner of a rather grim industrial park. Here Frank and his younger assistant, Sanh Phan, a Vietnamese refugee who had left his country on a wooden barge in the early 1980s, designed and built the oxygen- and nitrogen-generating machines, some of which weighed thousands of pounds and were double or triple the size of a standard refrigerator. Frank had hired Sanh a year after he arrived in the United States, through a Catholic charitable organization. Frank and Sanh had become close, and

Sanh soon referred to Frank as his uncle. There was only one other employee at On-Site Gas, an irascible secretary named Margaret who took orders from customers and managed the office.

But therein lay the fundamental problem. Even though Frank and Sanh had become masters at tuning and calibrating their creations and could produce oxygen and nitrogen that were 95 percent pure—a level of purity that was just about unheard of in the industry—there weren't that many customers. It turned out that Frank remained much more interested in inventing machines than actually selling them. He had hired an independent distributor to sell the machines for him, but that hadn't worked out either. If it weren't for Nancy's steady income as a nurse, the family wouldn't have been able to pay the mortgage on its home. Frank could just about pay the rent on On-Site's cramped offices—only fifty dollars a month—but the additional heating and hot water bills were sometimes beyond reach. In order not to freeze, Frank brought in electrical quartz heaters from home. Despite these challenges, even though Frank dearly loved his family, most Monday mornings he couldn't wait to get to work so he and Sanh could tinker with the machines. He could never quite believe that he had delivered on his adolescent pledge to have his own business, even if it was struggling.

Over the next decade, Frank more or less forgot about the miraculous blood clotting properties of zeolite. He became too busy with his family, his business, his parish. As the years passed, his hopes for what he had discovered about zeolite returned to what they had been before the patent: just an idea, or a theory, or a dream. Over time he grew more comfortable with the fact that the dream would never come to fruition and most likely would never exist outside the confines of his own mind.

But there were other times—typically late at night, before he went to bed, or as he sat in quiet reflection during Mass—when Frank would let his mind wander where he did not like to tread. He would think of the lost opportunities. In stopping bleeding, zeolite could potentially save thousands of lives—lives currently being lost in wars and car crashes. Shouldn't he be doing everything he could to get his discovery out into the world? Shouldn't he try to get it into the hands of those bleeding, suffering people and the ones who cared for them? But just as quickly as those discomfiting ideas came to Frank's mind, he would dismiss them. The idea was too staggering to consider. Besides, there were bills to pay, Little League games to attend, oxygen machines to build, further refinements to make with Sanh.

Still, Frank knew one thing for certain. He had proven that he could clot blood and that the caverns hidden inside zeolite absorbed water. His theory had been correct, and maybe that was enough. He had done what he had been trained to do as a mechanical engineer: to think of the body as a machine, bring a mechanical product into the body, and discover that it worked. Nobody else would even think to do such a thing. And in fact, Frank was the first person in recorded history to ever think of clotting blood by removing the water that it contained. Other scientists had conceived of ways to clot blood only through adding something to it, like more clotting proteins. Frank's genius was that he had gone in exactly the opposite direction from every other doctor and blood scientist. But all of this was unknown to Frank: working in near solitude, he had no awareness that he had changed a historic medical paradigm.

As the months turned into years and the years turned into decades, Frank maintained the routines of life in West Hartford, his thriving family, and his struggling business. He became inured to, and even comfortable with, the idea that he had solved this problem solely within the walls of his basement, and that no one—other than Nancy and some faceless person in the US Patent and Trademark Office—would ever know about it.

CHAPTER TWO

All Bleeding Stops Eventually

DURING THOSE THIRTY-SIX hours of operating on soldiers in the Forty-Sixth Combat Support Hospital at the edge of the Battle of Mogadishu, Major John Holcomb learned, in a way that few doctors ever do, the full import of the old medical saw that all bleeding stops eventually—which is to say that the patient heals, or the patient dies. Either way, the flow of blood comes to an end. In the aftermath of that experience, Holcomb decided that he, and the United States Army, were going to solve the problem of volume bleeding on the battlefield once and for all.

After all, Holcomb seemed the perfect candidate to solve this centuries-old medical mystery. He was brilliant, extraordinarily hardworking, and imbued with a powerful sense of certainty, which others, including his army superiors, found seductive. When he stated opinions, they often sounded like facts. Holcomb had a way of talking about medicine in definitive and forthright terms that everyone could understand. He was given to saying that even controversial treatments were "amazing" or "good for patients."

He came across as simultaneously smart and folksy, an impression reinforced by the pitch-perfect twang of his accent, which seemed to come from some ill-defined middle or southern part of America, the standard-issue way of speaking among army brass. He was tall and handsome and had a commanding, even swaggering, presence. He was also appealingly self-made, having grown up without wealth and attended tiny Centenary College of Louisiana in Shreveport, where he had been a biology major and a member of a fraternity, all while holding down three jobs. But Holcomb's greatest credential was that he had most formidably been "in the shit"—that is to say, in combat. He had served valiantly in warfare in a way that few doctors ever do. Within military medical culture, his harrowing experiences in Mogadishu were infinitely impressive, and, unlike the two doctors with whom he had served at the Forty-Sixth Combat Support Hospital, Holcomb did not appear to tire of speaking of them.

Holcomb was well aware that he had the opportunity to join a long and noble tradition of paradigm-shifting medical advances that had emerged from the cauldron of warfare. "Wars always cause improvements in trauma care," he told CNN. "The lessons that we learn in the military are going to apply ten- or a hundredfold to the civilian community." Or, as William Mayo, one of the founders of the famous Mayo Clinic, said more bluntly, "Medicine is the only victor in war." The examples were legion. The American Civil War brought about the first significant use of anesthesia. World War I led to the regular practice of blood transfusions. The field of chemotherapy was born after it was observed that soldiers exposed to mustard gas in World War I and II had lower white blood cell counts. White blood cells can divide quickly, and their suppression by mustard gas led scientists to the hypothesis, which proved correct, that mustard gas might kill rapidly dividing cancer cells as well. World War II saw the expanded use of antibiotics, specifically penicillin. Doctors in the Vietnam War pioneered the use of frozen blood products, which lasted months longer than fresh blood, and made extraordinary advances in burn care. It therefore seemed almost predestined that a similar medical miracle would emerge from the tragedy of Mogadishu.

Still, addressing traumatic blood loss in humans would be a daunting challenge. For centuries medicine had made very little progress in addressing one of the most fundamental problems of survival—keeping a sufficient amount of blood in the body so that a patient could stay alive. Blood, of course, transports oxygen from the lungs to the cells of the body, and it also provides cells with nutrients, transports hormones, and removes waste products. Blood is also critical to the regulation of body temperature; plasma—the clear, yellowish fluid that carries the blood cells—can both emit and absorb heat.

Blood is, of course, central to everything. In all cultures blood is an elemental concept, often synonymous with life itself. Goethe called it an "amiable juice," the book of Leviticus states that "the life of flesh is in the blood," the Bible mentions blood more than four hundred times, and one can't read more than a few pages in many of Shakespeare's plays without encountering the word *blood* or *bloodshed*. Blood is simultaneously largely invisible in our day-to-day lives and omnipresent in our cultures and consciousness. There remains something deeply mysterious about the liquid, and some of its basic facts are so mind-boggling that they don't even seem plausible. There are thirty trillion red blood cells in a person's body, and the circulatory system within each of us—of veins, arteries, and capillaries—is about sixty thousand miles long.

Given all this, it is odd that so little progress has been made in stanching bleeding, even after hundreds of years of effort. But trauma medicine is a particularly difficult area in which to make progress. Demetrios Demetriades of the University of Southern California, an internationally famous hematologist, said as much in a lecture in 2016 when he declared that "trauma is the least scientific of all major medical disciplines." There are many reasons for this, Demetriades explained, the primary one being that it is virtually impossible to conduct randomized clinical trials under the conditions of emergency medicine. How does one even ask a bleeding, possibly dying patient for informed consent? How do you explain to them the experimental treatment you are investigating? Often the patient is unconscious. And to make matters worse, Demetriades added, trauma surgeons, conversely, are quick "to adopt new flashy practices without any scientific evidence." There is a certain common sense to this: after all, surgeons are typically doers and practitioners—rather than researchers or scientists—who are temperamentally inclined to act rather than analyze and theorize. Perhaps this has to do with the intrinsic perilousness of the enterprise—the razor-thin margin between success and failure and the constant close proximity of death in an emergency operating room. The razor's edge gives doctors an understandable inclination to take risks and make decisions based on emotion and bias rather than evidence.

When Holcomb spoke at the RAND conference in Santa Monica in 2000, seven years after the events in Mogadishu, he showed images of ancient doctors using gauze on soldiers wounded in the Trojan War and photographs of gauze packets used in World Wars I and II. Holcomb was right when he said that nothing had changed in two millennia; the two treatments looked almost exactly the same. Indeed, for centuries trauma and military surgeons had been essentially powerless to do anything more than rely on the body's natural clotting processes to stop traumatic bleeding.

Doctors really had only two tools available, and both of them were rather primitive: manual pressure on the veins to stop blood from flowing out, and gauze in the wound to absorb blood and slow its movement. As long as the wound was not too massive, these tools were generally effective. The use of gauze and pressure generally bought the body critical time to build the fibrin clot, an insoluble protein that forms the major component of a blood clot. But both techniques were simply physical manipulations and did nothing intrinsically—biochemically—to speed up the natural clotting process. For all the advances that had been made across medicine, no drugs or supplements had been devised to stop streams of blood from flowing out of the traumatized body.

The cost of this failure was astounding. Bodily trauma is the fourth leading cause of death in the world, and half of those deaths are due to uncontrolled hemorrhage. In the United States, fifty thousand Americans a year bleed to death in hospitals and in the streets. Cruelly, trauma disproportionally affects the young, and it is the leading cause of death for Americans under the age of forty-five.

Upon returning to the United States from Mogadishu, Holcomb became a researcher at the army's Institute of Surgical Research in San Antonio, Texas—the ISR, as it is universally known. With a staff of many hundreds of doctors and researchers, the ISR is one of six major research laboratories across the country within the army's Medical Command and is the only one dedicated solely to improving the care of combat casualties. (Other institutes have similarly focused areas, such as the National Institute of Allergy and Infectious Diseases, the US Army Medical Research Institute of Chemical Defense in Maryland, and the US Army Research Institute of Environmental Medicine in Massachusetts.) The ISR had begun modestly in 1943 as a branch of Halloran General

Hospital on Staten Island, New York, with just twelve employees. The institute moved to Texas four years later, and in the 1950s its focus largely turned to the treatment of thermal injury, in anticipation of causalities from nuclear weapons. Under the leadership of its director, Dr. Basil Pruitt, the ISR became known as "the Army's Burn Center" and was internationally recognized for its excellence in this area. But for all its prominence, the ISR remained a somewhat mysterious and murky institution. Few of its activities were publicized, and its research studies were typically reported in a medical journal of mixed reputation, the *Journal of Trauma*. This journal seemed at times to have erratic editorial standards, and at times an unusually narrow group of contributors, many of them army doctors. For example, some articles by contributors, including those coauthored by Holcomb, were received and accepted within a day or two, an atypical practice in the world of medical journals.

While the institute's clinical focus was theoretically the entire spectrum of care for those wounded in combat, it was not until Holcomb's arrival that the ISR undertook significant work in the area of traumatic bleeding. Holcomb threw himself into the problem, writing multiple grants to develop blood clotting products and publishing prolifically about them. From 1998 through 2008, his name and byline came to dominate the journal. Holcomb published many dozens of articles, the vast majority of them coauthored, in the *Journal of Trauma*.

He rose with remarkable speed at the Institute of Surgical Research. By 1999 he was director of trauma research, and by 2002 he was commander of the entire institute. He had barely turned forty. In his new position, Holcomb was supervising hundreds of doctors, some of them two decades his senior. The hierarchical nature of the institute empowered him to make bold, decisive, and often unilateral decisions. "One of the things that makes [the institute] is that it has a commander, it doesn't have a director," said Colonel Shawn Nessen, who succeeded Holcomb in the role. "Command is everything in the Army, and commanders can make things happen." Indeed, Holcomb later quipped that his leadership philosophy was that "a colonel and his memo can do almost anything."

To John Holcomb and his fellow army researchers, as well as hematologists working in hospitals and labs around the world, it was axiomatic that if you were going to fundamentally solve the problem of traumatic bleeding, there were only two possible approaches. Either you had to turbocharge the body's natural clotting cascade by enhancing the thirteen clotting proteins, or you had to bioengineer a bandage loaded with chemicals that would strengthen the fibrin clot. Both techniques were expensive and complex. To be effective, genetically created (or naturally occurring, from animals) clotting proteins had to be heavily concentrated, twenty to one hundred times more potent than in their natural state. Such clotting proteins typically must be extracted from genetically modified animals—pigs, cows, hamsters—and the production of even a single treatment for a patient could take a year. They also had to be safe, which meant multiple rounds of testing and purification. Earlier attempts at using engineered clotting proteins had led to patients contracting serious diseases like hepatitis that were transmitted from animal to human.

Human blood is about 50 percent plasma, which is the watery part. The other half of blood—the solid part—is made up of platelets and red and white blood cells. When a blood vessel is injured, three events occur in rapid succession. First, the vessel contracts so less blood will leak out. Second, platelets—tiny, round, colorless cell fragments—travel to the injured area to form a plug. There, the platelets release chemicals to attract more platelets. Then thirteen distinct clotting factors, each one a discrete protein, are activated in sequence, like a row of falling dominoes. The clotting factors travel to and bind with the platelets at the wound site to form an even bigger plug, the fibrin clot, which creates a tighter and more durable mesh, sealing the wound. Once the clot is complete, additional proteins are activated that prevent it from growing larger than it needs to be. When the wound is healed and the clot is no longer needed, the fibrin is cut up into pieces and the fragments are excreted in urine.

It is a remarkable and intricate process, and despite the protestations of some hematologists, it is one that is still not completely understood. But as miraculous as it is, there is a limit to what the body's natural clotting processes can achieve. The process can be fatally slow and inefficent. If the wound is too large or too deep, the body can't clot quickly enough. Time is of the essence. The average person has only about a gallon and a half of blood. Lose half of that amount over a few hours, and the patient is most likely dead. With massive blood loss, a "lethal triad" ocurs, a potentially fatal combination of hypothermia (low body temperature), acidosis (high levels of acid in blood and other body fluids), and coagulopathy (impaired clot formation). As blood continues to flow from the body, these three factors build viciously on one another: blood loss causes lower body temperature; lower body temperature impairs clotting functions; impaired clotting results in increased lactic acid in the blood; and excess lactic acid leads to decreased heart performance, causing low body temperature. And on and on until the patient goes into shock and dies.

But there's a reason blood clotting is slow and inefficent. It has to be. While blood clotting in the right places is essential to survival, clotting in the wrong places can kill. Blood clots, so lifesaving at the site of a wound, can be deadly when they travel elsewhere in the body. A blood clot that breaks loose can pass, via the bloodstream, to the lungs, heart, or brain, where it can stop blood flow in these vital organs. A blood clot in the artery of a lung causes a pulmonary embolism. Clots in the arteries of the brain lead to strokes, and in those of the heart to heart attacks. Death as a result of blood clots is surprisingly common: up to a hundred thousand Americans die from clots each year.

So there was a reason it took two millenia to stop traumatic bleeding. It is a messy, perilous, even ugly business. Clot too little and a patient will die of his wounds, but clot too much and the patient will die of another cause.

Starting in 1997, at the Institute of Surgical Research, John Holcomb was at the center of a collaboration with the American Red Cross to create a bandage to strengthen the fibrin seal. He wrote eight grants totaling hundreds of thousands of dollars for the project. The idea was to produce a bandage four inches square and loaded with the freeze-dried clotting proteins fibrinogen and thrombin. The bandage would be pressed onto a wound and held there for two minutes, during which time its materials would dissolve into the bloodstream. The fibrinogen and thrombin were extracted from the milk of genetically altered pigs raised on a farm in Blacksburg, Virginia.

The bandage was actually based on an old idea. During both World Wars, surgeons devastated by mounting casualties desperately sought new ways to stop bleeding. They dried blood and sprinkled it on wounds to encourage clotting. They sealed wounds with fibrin glue, fibrin sheet foam, and fibrin powder—materials that were mass-produced from plasma—but the projects were withdrawn in 1946 because the techniques could transmit hepatitis to soldiers. But fibrin does have one massive advantage. It does not course through the body like other clotting agents but is activated directly at the wound site, where it contorts itself into a fine, interlacing mesh that traps blood cells and sticks fiercely to a wound to form a scab.

Early reviews of the army and Red Cross bandage, even before it was finished, were ecstatic. It was as if everyone agreed that the bandage's designers were on the verge of a momentous discovery. "This is really the first significant advance in emergency treatment to stem blood loss in about three thousand years," said Dr. William Drohan, director of the Red Cross plasma research lab. "This fibrin bandage is the single most important advance in technology for the military," enthused Admiral Michael Cowen, surgeon general to the Joint Chiefs of Staff. Holcomb himself said that the bandage was going to transform emergency medicine. "As it becomes FDA approved, surgeons, paramedics, and emergency doctors will use it in ways we haven't even thought of yet." He and his Red Cross colleagues estimated their invention would generate $400 million a year in sales and predicted that the bandages would be carried in police cars, ambulances, and everyday first-aid kits.

The national media endorsed what seemed like a near coronation of the medical breakthrough. Even though the bandage was still years away from actually being fielded, the following headlines about the project appeared in the mid-to-late-1990s:

"Stopping Bleeding with Biologic Glue," Washington Post *(August 6, 1996)*

"New Bandage Creates Instant Blood Clots," Knight Ridder (March 3, 1999)

"New Bandage Could Avert Thousands of Deaths," New York
Times *(March 9, 1999)*
"Hope of Survival Wrapped in a Simple Bandage," Washington Post
(May 12, 1999)
"Scientists Using Blood Proteins to Create Lifesaving Bandage,"
Washington Post *(June 14, 1999)*

Indeed, as the bandage was developed and tested over the
next few years, it was shown to slow arterial bleeding in animals
within fifteen to sixty seconds, reducing blood loss by between 50
and 85 percent. But there was a catch. The process of developing the bandage was so complex and lengthy that each bandage
cost approximately $1,000. Early testing also indicated that the
bandage was flimsy, easily sloughing off the wound when used in
the field. Lieutenant Commander Joseph Dacorta, a counterpart
of Holcomb's in the navy, declined the army's request to support
the project. Dacorta thought there was a good chance that viruses
from the animals' proteins could spread to humans. He was also
concerned about the bandage's extraordinary expense, knowing
that $1,000 a bandage was a figure one would have to multiply
by more than a million in order to supply every soldier with the
product. And as a former combat medic, he wondered about how
the bandage would be adequately stored. Fibrin is essentially a
protein, and proteins degrade over time, requiring refrigeration.
How would such a product be incorporated into the supply chain to
the battlefield? What was its shelf life? He predicted—correctly—
that the FDA would never approve it.

But Holcomb and the ISR were undeterred by such consider-
ations. In fact, the hunt to find the ultimate blood clotting agent
had ramped up even further by the late 1990s with the publication
of Mark Bowden's *Black Hawk Down,* a meticulously researched

book about the Battle of Mogadishu, which was turned into a hit Hollywood movie in 2001. The climax of the movie focused on the story of Corporal Jamie Smith, who had grown up in northern New Jersey and graduated from high school—where he had played football and lacrosse and been a Boy Scout—only three years before the Battle of Mogadishu. His father had been an army captain in Vietnam, and Jamie Smith had wanted to be an Army Ranger his whole life. As described in *Black Hawk Down*, during the opening salvos of the battle, Smith crouched behind a small tin shed only ten yards from the road where the first Black Hawk lay prone. Bullets flew all around him, seemingly coming from every direction, flying through the shed. Smith stepped out into the street and got on his knee to begin shooting in the direction of a Somali man across the street. In the first moments after being hit, Smith seemed surprised, and then he fell to the ground and rolled to his side. Two of Smith's fellow soldiers, one a medic, dashed out into the street from their protected positions and, somehow avoiding gunfire, dragged him into the safety of a courtyard. The medic immediately got to work. Blood spouted, fountain-like, from Smith's upper leg. The bullet had severed his femoral artery, one of the largest in the body, buried deep in the fleshiest part of the thigh. In a proper hospital emergency room, Smith's wound would have been very serious but treatable; stopping the bleeding, even as voluminous as it was, would simply be a matter of cutting open the thigh and pinching off the artery. But in the middle of a street battle with only his kit bag, the medic couldn't reach the site of Smith's wound to clamp the artery. With no other recourse, he used gauze on the wound, but it only marginally slowed the blood racing out of Smith's fading body.

If Smith was to survive, he needed to be evacuated to John Holcomb's Forty-Sixth Combat Support Hospital, where the artery could be tied on a surgeon's table. Over the din of grenades and automatic weapons fire, the medic radioed for a medevac by helicopter. The request was denied; the commanding officer said words to the effect that, given the intensity of the battle, saving Smith's life would incur too much risk to the lives of other soldiers. The medic could only give Jamie Smith morphine. As he faded away, Smith prayed with the medic, asking him to tell his family that he loved them. At the very end, Smith hyperventilated, and then his heart stopped beating. The medic tried CPR and injected drugs directly into Smith's heart, to no avail.

The filmed version of *Black Hawk Down* is relentlessly violent from start to finish, and Smith's death, which provides the climax of the movie, is portrayed as being particularly pointless and barbaric, almost medieval. In a kind of pornographic detail, the scene revealed the army's inability to take care of its own. Audiences were left to wonder, Why couldn't the army, with all its money and resources and prestige, help a man who had suffered a relatively simple wound? Why couldn't the US Army save a brave soldier's life?

But Holcomb believed the Red Cross bandage would solve all of that. In *JAMA: The Journal of the American Medical Association*, in 1998, he wrote of the bandage, "When fielded in final form, we see this as a forward projection of advanced hemorrhage control outside the operating room, providing urban and military casualties rapid, definitive hemorrhage control." But after being beta tested by special operations forces, the bandage was used in combat during the war on terror in Afghanistan only once. That sole use was successful, but the bandage would prove unstable, flaking off the wound and literally falling apart. The entire years-long project was summarily scrapped.

If Holcomb was disappointed, he never showed it. Instead, imbued with his inveterate optimism and drive, he had already thrown himself into finding another agent to clot blood. In 2001, as the nation tilted toward war, Dr. Kenton Gregory, a chemical engineer and physician at the Oregon Medical Laser Center, began investigating the hemostatic properties of shrimp shells after a member of his staff told him that for centuries Chinese fishermen had used shrimp shells on their cracked and bleeding hands, rubbing the material into their cuts and abrasions. Gregory and his colleagues looked into a chemical called chitosan, found in the outer shells of shrimp, as well as other crustaceans, which they believed had the capacity to stanch blood. Gregory conducted early tests on a bandage that he impregnated with the shrimp-derived chitosan, and the results were promising. Gregory called the bandage, and the company eventually created to produce it, HemCon—short for *hemorrhage control*.

John Holcomb and his colleagues at the Institute of Surgical Research heard about the HemCon bandage and flew to Oregon, and observed as the prototype chitosan pads were pressed onto the bleeding arteries of pigs. He and his team from the institute were impressed. "We were just as skeptical as always, and maybe more skeptical because we already knew about some chitosan dressings that didn't work," said Anthony Pusateri, who led the army's hemostasis program under Holcomb. (*Hemostatis* is the technical term for the stopping of bleeding or hemorrhage.) "But this one, even in its early prototypes, did a phenomenal job of controlling hemorrhage." Holcomb would soon become an evangelist for HemCon. He would later say about the bandage, with his characteristic effusiveness, "It has no known side effects, the performance is amazing in every study we have developed, and the reports from people who actually use the product have been positive."

Many in the army believed HemCon was going to do what the Red Cross fibrin bandage had failed to do: solve traumatic bleeding on the battlefield once and for all. Even though the second round of testing showed less convincing results, army medicine, led by Holcomb, immediately went about pouring tens of millions of dollars into the production of the HemCon bandage. The later bankruptcy papers for the HemCon company, filed in 2013, revealed that it had received a total of $76 million in military grants, which included funding to purchase HemCon bandages, $19 million in private financings with outside investors, and $37 million in bank debt. But for now, Holcomb and the United States Army seemed convinced they were now on the cusp of solving one of the medical mysteries of the ages. It never once seemed to occur to them that perhaps somebody already had.

CHAPTER THREE

The Salesman with Nothing to Sell

TWO YEARS BEFORE scientists across the country in Oregon were beginning their work on HemCon, on a fall day in 1999 a man named Bart Gullong drove his ten-year-old brown Ford Thunderbird into the parking lot of Paradise Pizza in New Britain, Connecticut. He was about to have lunch with a fifty-seven-year-old inventor and mechanical engineer named Frank Hursey, whom he had never met. The meeting was about a business opportunity at Frank's company, On-Site Gas Systems, and possibly a job—which Gullong desperately needed. He had been unemployed for a year.

Bart looked at himself in the rearview mirror. Looking back at him was a fifty-one-year-old man with sharp features, a salt-and-pepper goatee, and chestnut hair rakishly swept back over his forehead. Bart did not particularly like the man he saw. For the last fifteen years, he'd felt bruised and bitter, seething with unfulfilled promise. He had been an elite rower in prep school and college, and immediately after college he had become a rowing coach.

The first season he ever coached—working with a high school team in its first year of existence—he had brought home the state championship. The next year, Bart became the men's and women's rowing coach at Connecticut College, a prestigious liberal arts college, where he recruited future Olympians and transformed the program in one year. By age twenty-five, he was part of the small group of coaches who had won the US national women's rowing championship. At age thirty, after becoming dean of students at a college on Long Island, he became an entrepreneur, starting his own video game business and inventing a speedometer for rowing shells and selling it to a sports instrumentation company. In the late 1970s, on a flight to Houston, Bart was seated next to a hiring director for NASA. By the time the plane touched down in Texas, he had been hired as a consultant to work on the computer/pilot interface in the design of the first space shuttle. Bart had done all of these things on the strength of a degree in English literature. But the degree was not entirely irrelevant; from great literature Bart had learned that he could use stories to sell products, influence customers, and, not least, promote himself.

But for the last fifteen years, Bart's life had followed an entirely different narrative arc: he'd lived in the raucous Hamptons of Long Island, bouncing among women and stumbling through a bad first marriage. He had spent more time than he liked to admit exploring the Hamptons bar scene. To get by he captained luxury boats for wealthy clients, sometimes spending entire seasons sailing around the Caribbean islands. He also flipped houses and sold yachts, hating almost every moment of it. When he began to hate himself too, he realized that he had had enough and moved back to boring central Connecticut with his four-year-old daughter and second wife. Connecticut, then and now, was known as "the Land of Steady Habits," and it was where Bart had grown up. He thought the state, with its broad reputation for propriety and lack of excess, at least when compared to the roaring Hamptons, would be as good a place as any to straighten himself out and provide a healthier and simply more normal place for his daughter to grow up.

Over the course of the last twelve months, he had sent out hundreds of résumés. Not one company had responded. Increasingly desperate, Bart had contacted Frank Hursey, whom he was about to meet in the pizza place, after reading Frank's ad in the *Hartford Courant* seeking a business partner or investor in his company. Something in the notice intrigued Bart—something about gas-generating systems. But with his dwindling bank account, Bart was hardly in a position to invest. If indeed Hursey was going to insist on some kind of financial relationship, Bart would have to get the money through a second mortgage on his house. Still, something inside Bart told him that he should meet with Hursey; he sensed that something about what Hursey was doing seemed interesting.

In middle age, Bart had begun to think of himself as a salesman with nothing to sell. He had spent a lot of the last six months sitting around the house, depressed and angry at himself, mindlessly writing barbecue recipes, which had become an obsession. He had recently been turned down for a job selling used cars at a dealership on the side of a bleak highway, and another as a promoter for a DJ business that catered to nightclubs and parties in Hartford. In fact, before he answered Frank's posting, he was just about to give up on sales entirely. He was thinking about getting his license as a commercial long-distance trucker. At least that would get him out of the house. He had partied his life away and become a loser, a fucking modern-day Willy Loman.

Enough, enough, he thought. *I've got a meeting. Get into salesman mode. Crush them with your handshake and your confidence.*

Inside the restaurant, Bart immediately spotted Hursey in a booth in the back. Frank was just as he had described himself on the phone the day before, "slight and Irish looking." Bart introduced himself and sat down. After the two ordered, Frank began to talk hesitantly, almost shyly, about his company. On-Site Gas Systems made oxygen generators for medical and industrial purposes, he said. Frank invented the machines and constructed them by hand. He explained that his company had only two other employees and had not grown in ten years, and there were months in which he struggled financially. It quickly became clear to Bart why. Even in their brief conversation, Bart saw that Frank cared mainly about the minute details of how the machines operated and considered the actual selling of his products either tedious or irrelevant. Bart also saw that Frank was fixated on a mineral, zeolite, which he employed to separate oxygen and nitrogen.

Frank actually had not talked about his discovery about zeolite to anyone for some time, but for some reason he felt comfortable with Bart and thought that he might understand his excitement. He decided to take a chance on Bart. Frank excitedly told him about the caverns in zeolite and said he'd once done an experiment on a mouse that immediately stopped the animal's bleeding. This did not sound at all credible to Bart. In fact, as the lunch went on, Bart began to fear that little about Frank was credible. But at the same time, Bart couldn't help but be intrigued by the possibilities. For all his shortcomings at sales, Frank certainly appeared to be a unique inventor, perhaps even a brilliant one. What if he had someone by his side who could actually explain what the machines did and cared about selling them? Maybe this was the opportunity Bart had been seeking for decades.

After lunch, Frank invited Bart to the premises of On-Site Gas, a quarter mile away. Frank had certainly implied that his business was not thriving, but Bart didn't realize how bad things actually were until he saw the offices in the forlorn back corner of an industrial park. Inside was a dusty reception area with two adjoining offices, the walls lined with dark fake wood paneling. The desks were heaped with papers, and the chairs and file cabinets looked like cast-off World War II–era furniture, which in fact they were. Frank introduced Bart to his office manager, Margaret, who seemed to take an immediate dislike to him. The whole thing was depressing.

But then Frank showed him the oxygen machines in the workshop. They were towering, boxy consoles weighing thirteen hundred pounds each, with all kinds of gauges and instruments attached to them. At this point Bart didn't quite know how they worked, but he could tell—it was obvious—they were masterfully engineered and constructed. Frank introduced Bart to Sanh and explained that while he designed the machines, he and Sanh built them together. Sanh, immediately after meeting Bart, asked him plaintively, "Can you take our company where we need to go?"

"Yes I can," Bart said. "Absolutely." It wasn't a total lie; it was clear to Bart that for all the shabbiness around him, these two men in an unknown corner of Connecticut were producing something extraordinary.

Frank invited Bart into his cramped office, where he proudly showed Bart the company's website, which was populated with stick figure animations, and also its relatively new logo. It featured the slogan *On-Site Gas Systems, Celebrating Our 10th Year*. Bart couldn't help but think, *You've been around for ten years and this is as far as you've gotten?*

When they got down to business, Frank said he had changed his mind: based on painful experiences he had in the past, he had decided he was no longer looking for a business partner or investor.

Bart was slightly taken aback, but said, "That's fine. How about I come work for you?"

"But I don't have any money to hire anyone," Frank said.

They talked awkwardly around the issue for a while. But in those moments Bart decided that he couldn't leave the meeting without having some kind of deal in place. He couldn't return home that night and not be able to tell his wife, Linda, that he had some kind of a plan. He needed to tell her that he was going to take care of their family.

Bart asked, "What do you pay your distributor to sell the machines?"

"Twenty-five percent," Frank replied.

"How about I sell the machines, and I will take the twenty-five percent," Bart said. "In other words, I will become your in-house distributor. You won't have anything to lose."

"Wow, I guess in that case I wouldn't," Frank said.

Bart said, "I will make you a wealthy man in one year's time, Frank."

Frank laughed awkwardly at the absurdity of the thought.

Nonetheless they shook hands on the deal. Of course, Bart knew he had just agreed to take a job with no salary or health insurance. That part might be hard to explain to Linda. But in the end it was surprisingly easy to say yes to Frank. Even though they had just met, Bart found something pure, even inspiring, about him. He liked his earnest, gentle manner. After fifteen years in the Hamptons, something about Frank's lack of guile gave Bart hope.

But there was one thing that concerned him. It was this talk of zeolite, and specifically how it could clot blood. "It works great," Frank said, "I know it does." That sounded like science fiction to Bart. How could an obscure mineral used in machines also stop people from bleeding? Who would even think to put such a thing in their body? And why would a guy whose business was making oxygen generators spend so much time talking about blood clotting? It made Frank seem like an easily distracted crackpot, which Bart surely hoped he wasn't. His future depended on it.

Later, as he drove home, Bart realized there was another thing about the meeting that he didn't like. Frank's offices reminded Bart of his father's workplace, which was not pleasant to remember. Bart's father had been a personnel manager at an engineering firm not far from On-Site Gas, and Bart had occasionally visited him at work. These were unhappy occasions. Bart's father was a sullen World War II vet who seemed to take special pleasure in verbally torturing his son. "You thought you were a man, but you're just a foolish little boy," he would say as Bart shot up during adolescence. Nothing Bart did was ever good enough. Once Bart's crew performed brilliantly in a six boat race, finishing a close second. In the moments after the race, his father congratulated him, but on the ride home he said, "Couldn't you have won?" Bart had grown up believing there was something sadistic about his father, some deep hatred inside him. It was always left to his mother, typically gracious and warm, to smooth things over.

For his part, Frank was concerned that Bart was just some fast-talking salesperson. Frank had hired a number of slick salesmen over the years and been burned every time. He also had lingering suspicions that Bart was some kind of rich kid, a preppy. Frank had grown up in a poor and depressed household, while Bart's family had had a summer cottage in Old Saybrook, half a mile from where Katharine Hepburn lived, and spent the summers sailing the Long Island Sound. Bart had gone to a boarding school, of all things. As Frank got to know Bart better, he would learn that Bart's mother, a high school teacher, had a PhD in classics and had attended Bates, Trinity, and Harvard. All of this seemed a little foreign or off-putting to Frank. And so, before fully committing to hiring Bart, Frank engaged a private detective to see if he could find anything on him. The private eye tailed Bart for a day or so and even went through Bart's garbage cans. The only things that turned up were parking tickets.

Over the course of the next five months, Bart learned everything he could about how the machines functioned and promoted them to anyone who would listen. But he didn't make a single sale, and therefore was not paid a single dollar. Linda was concerned and becoming impatient. It had now been a year and a half since Bart had generated any income. But in the sixth month, Bart finally closed a deal. It was not for one or two of the machines, as Frank had been selling them for years, but for one hundred of them, to Monro Mufflers. Bart and Frank had figured out that the oxygen generated by the machines could be used to power an intense flame capable of cutting through metal, and Bart had sold the idea to Monro as an efficient means of excising old mufflers from cars. It was a $300,000 sale, and it turned out that it would be the first of many big deals. There were more sales to muffler companies, and in the next year, 2000, the floodgates opened. Bart redesigned and restructured the On-Site Gas website around specific keywords, and inquiries started pouring in from all over the country: New York City, Indianapolis, Little Rock, Minneapolis. It made all the difference that Bart could explain, in ways that were simple and accessible, how the machines functioned, and, most importantly, what they could actually do for the customer. He built a display box containing wooden balls representing individual molecules to show how Frank's pressure swing technology—the apparatus that drove the machines—worked. Bart studied the airline schedules out of Hartford and learned that as long as he didn't travel farther west than Houston, he could leave Connecticut early in the morning and be home in time to make up a story to tell his daughter at bedtime. Soon he was on the road two, three, even four days a week. After so many years of unproductive activity, Bart found it exhilarating, particularly when most trips resulted in sales, often big sales. Soon Frank and Bart were meeting every Friday to go over orders and strategy and review their daily and weekly logs, which they called a "booked-to-build" system. It was their bible. But there was a price to pay for all the evident progress the company was making. Bart became torn up with guilt about missing most of Sarah's childhood. He felt he was not living up to his responsibility as a parent, and it began to torment him.

Within a year and a half of being hired, Bart and Frank were both suddenly making money—real money, hundreds of thousands of dollars a year—and Bart was making so much on commission that he was earning considerably more than Frank. They agreed on a handshake deal to reduce Bart's commission in exchange for partial ownership of the company. Profits were significant enough that Frank moved On-Site into an impressive new facility: the entire first floor of a large, well-appointed building with plush offices in front and a large workshop with twenty-foot ceilings in back, set on a hill looking over a busy turnpike just south of Hartford. They hired ten, then twenty employees, mainly Bosnian refugees whom Frank contacted through Catholic Charities. Frank paid above-market wages and liked to hire people who were fleeing difficult circumstances. Gradually and ineffably, Bart felt his sense of self-worth returning; for the first time in years, he could look at himself in the mirror without cringing.

On a beautiful morning in September 2001, two planes flew into the World Trade Center in New York City. Five days after the attacks, Frank and his son drove to New York City and donated medical oxygen generators to the New York City firefighters in downtown Manhattan, to be used to revive them after smoke inhalation. In the wake of 9/11, Frank thought there might be a need for his long-lost zeolite blood clotting idea, and he had the mineral tested for basic safety standards—to make sure it wasn't poisonous or toxic—at a lab in Springfield, Massachusetts. Around this time, Bart, who daily scoured the internet for business opportunities, came across a solicitation from the air force. Bart had been targeting military solicitations, knowing the Pentagon's budget would surge in the tense days after 9/11. The air force had issued a request for proposals to develop portable surgical centers that could be set up as close to the battlefield as possible and used to perform basic operations on wounded soldiers and stabilize them before they were brought to larger facilities. The centers, called Forward Resuscitative Surgical Systems, would have to be sufficiently small to be transported in two Humvees and minimal enough to be assembled in less than an hour. The system called for a medical oxygen machine to deliver thirty liters of oxygen per minute. Bart realized that such a machine would essentially be a vastly scaled-down version of what Frank and Sanh had been building for years. He excitedly brought the opportunity to Frank. Frank was uncharacteristically negative. Designing such equipment, Frank said, would require reducing his oxygen generators to three hundred pounds, a quarter of their current size. The machines, Frank explained, were governed by the laws of physics and needed to be a certain size to function properly.

Bart said, "But this is our one shot. We've got to do this." Bart was thrilled with the financial turnaround that the company was experiencing but had believed all along that if On-Site was really going to take off, they needed to get in with the military. Over the next six weeks, Bart first persuaded Frank to agree to the project, and then Sanh, Bart, and Frank worked hundreds of hours of overtime to build a semifunctional prototype by the air force's upcoming deadline. They called their machine the POGS, short for Portable Oxygen Generating System. Bart took on the role of the coach he had once been, badgering Sanh and even Frank to push themselves harder, night after late night. Sanh, in particular, chafed at Bart's aggressive directions, and said one night that he wasn't going to work on the project anymore. Bart said, "OK, then, fuck it." Sanh, whose English was not perfect, thought that Bart had said, "Fuck you." They almost came to blows and had to be separated by Frank. Bart towered over both Frank and Sanh, but he ultimately backed off. By the deadline, the team had built a complex but still crude machine that barely matched the solicitation's specifications. Bart asked, for credibility's sake, that it be painted an army combat green. Not picking up on the nuances of the request, Sanh painted the POGS machine a bright shamrock color. Bart took to calling the mortifying contraption the Jolly Green Giant.

On the morning that the military reps arrived, Frank splurged on coffee and doughnuts in an effort to be hospitable. As the officials stood by, Bart and Sanh rolled the Jolly Green Giant unsteadily toward them. Bart half expected the thing to topple over. One of the air force reps said, "We didn't think you'd actually build one. All the other companies just drew up plans. We can't believe you actually did this!" On-Site Gas was awarded the $400,000 contract.

After the award, the project—for reasons that were never made clear to Bart and Frank—was transferred from the air force to the purview of the marines. Bart and On-Site Gas were assigned to a senior enlisted officer, Master Chief Thomas Eagles of the Marine Corps Warfighting Laboratory in Quantico, Virginia, who would serve as the project lead. Eagles, or Tommy, as he asked to be called, was in charge of medical technology for the entire Marine Corps. Bart and Tommy began speaking weekly, even daily, on the phone. Eagles often referred to "the kid in the ditch," by which he meant the terrified young marine left alone to die in some dark corner of the battlefield. "I work for the kid in the ditch," Eagles said. "I don't know how many marines and sailors I helped save, but I remember everyone I lost." Indeed, Eagles had been such a "kid" himself, coming from a poor family in upstate New York, who had been shot on four separate occasions in Vietnam, once when he had run into an open field to save a wounded Vietnamese child. He never stopped talking about "the kid in the ditch," and he seemed to want to use his remaining time in the service to do everything in his power to get the right equipment to marines in combat.

Bart learned that Eagles was probably the most decorated navy medic in American medical history. He had flown 221 combat missions in Vietnam and won an extraordinary three Purple Hearts, four Silver Stars, and the Distinguished Flying Cross—surely the only medic to ever win such a medal. He received it for helping to land a helicopter after the pilot had been killed. Eagles called it "the worst helicopter landing in history." He first came to Vietnam as a Catholic monk in 1963 and was one of the last Americans to leave the country, airlifted off the roof of the US embassy on the last day of the war, in 1975. Eagles was constantly laughing and joking. "My ass has been chewed out by generals so many times I can't sit down" was a common utterance. He would ask, "What do you call a marine with an IQ of 160?" "A platoon," he would answer. Eagles's other signature phrase was "the fucking brass." He hated the fucking brass. Despite his status, Eagles was still an enlisted man—not an officer. However, Bart learned from others—because Eagles would never even bring up such things—that as a master chief, Eagles was one of the most senior enlisted members in the entire Marine Corps.

Tommy and Bart talked for months on the phone before actually meeting in person. Bart always pictured him, given his title and his exploits—and his made-for-Hollywood last name—as a strapping, bursting-at-the-seams, Sergeant Rock kind of figure, even though Eagles surely would now be well over sixty years old. As the Portable Oxygen Generating System was getting ready for deployment, Bart was invited to Quantico, the fifty-five-thousand-acre home of the marines in Virginia, to attend a product demonstration of military technologies by the contractors who had built and developed them. The event was going to be held in a massive tent and amount to a dog and pony show for military brass. Bart was so intimidated by the prospect of meeting Eagles that he tried to get in the best shape he could before the demonstration. He starved himself and lost fifteen pounds in a month. On the day of the event, he wore a particularly elegant beige suit. When he finally got to Quantico, which was teeming with contractors showing off their wares, Bart looked for Tommy. He was directed to a smallish man with a pot-belly and sporting a cane and a fedora. Eagles had been suffering for years from the effects of Agent Orange.

Around this time—early 2002—Bart and his wife saw the movie *Black Hawk Down*, which had just come out. Bart was overcome watching the scene of Jamie Smith's death, which was featured in agonizing detail. It had been a few years since Frank had talked much about his zeolite invention, although Bart knew that Frank had recently done some basic safety testing on the product. But as Bart watched the movie, he thought: *What if we—Frank and I—could save the next Jamie Smith?* What if Frank was onto something with that zeolite idea? You never knew with Frank; part of him was a genius, and part of him was...well, you just didn't know. It was great they were getting major contracts, but Bart wanted more. He wanted to make up for all that lost time in his forties.

One day on the phone Eagles was complaining about "the fucking brass," as was his wont. Eagles said, "I have this bullshit thing I have to do this week. The fucking brass want me to take part in the blood clotting trial. You know the military is always looking out for the next hemostatic agent, and these things never work...they are just a big waste of time..."

Bart immediately piped up. "You know, Tommy, we might have something that clots blood. Frank has been talking for years about..."

Eagles snapped back, uncharacteristically sharp, "Look, you're doing a great job with the oxygen generator. Don't screw it up by chasing after the next thing. Don't try and be like all these other contractors on the gravy train." Indeed, Bart had seen dozens of just such contractors fawning over Eagles at the demonstration event at Quantico.

Bart said, "Tommy, I have no idea if it works or not. I just know Frank said it does." Eagles didn't want to hear anything more about it. He got off the phone quickly. But a week later, Eagles called back. He said that one of the companies in the upcoming trial had unexpectedly canceled and that he could possibly get Bart's product on the docket—*if Bart was really sure he had something*. Bart and Frank FedExed a sample of ground-up zeolite to Quantico, but not before putting it in the microwave first because Frank said it would work better if the mineral was heated, causing a vacuum to develop within the rock as it cooled. Bart also bought a food sealer at Target for $175 to package the zeolite in a vacuum-sealed packet in an attempt to preserve the granules in their new state and at least make their submission look semiprofessional. They sent one hundred grams of the mineral—the equivalent of about one cup of sugar. Based on Frank's fairly limited knowledge of how zeolite actually worked, they wrote up simple directions: sprinkle zeolite into the wound, wait for the clot to form, then irrigate to get rid of the excess granular material.

The trial was sponsored by the Office of Naval Research, or ONR, whose mission is to provide new technologies for the navy and the Marine Corps. The ONR, however, had a relatively small budget, and compared to similar departments in the army, it seemed to fly under the radar. Some staffers had taken to calling ONR "the Brain Trust You Never Heard Of." ONR was organized around departments, or "codes," as they were called, which covered everything from aircraft to ships to antisubmarine warfare to weapons. It was Code 34—the Department of Warfighter Performance— that sponsored the trial. The Warfighter Performance Department was tasked with enhancing warfighter effectiveness and efficiency through bioengineered and biorobotic systems and medical and behavioral technologies. One of the program officers was Dr. Michael Given, a mild-mannered fifty-five-year-old pharmacologist who had been in the army in Vietnam as part of a recon platoon setting up ambushes and operating mainly at night. He was a forward observer, directing artillery and calling in air strikes. Most of the members of his platoon were killed. However, Given rarely spoke about his time in Vietnam. He was self-effacing to the extreme and preferred to talk about his work, his family, and his struggling golf game.

A week later, Bart and Frank were invited to the navy hospital in Bethesda for a pretrial meeting. But Bart alone decided to go. Frank wasn't much up for travel; increasingly, when he wasn't at On-Site, his life revolved around the home. He was devoted to his wife, Nancy, who had been diagnosed with diabetes at a young age. It had not stopped her from a full and rewarding career as a nurse, but gradually she was starting to slow down. Besides, Bart and Frank agreed that

Bart was much better suited to being the outward face of the company.

Bart arrived at the 9:00 a.m. meeting, having taken an early flight from Hartford. The meeting was run by Eagles's colleague Lieutenant Commander Joseph Dacorta of the navy, a compact man of medium height and build. Each of the other men in the conference room—there were about eight of them—introduced himself as a PhD or MD at a biotech or medical company, and they all seemed to know each other. They were all working on some type of blood clotting agent, and many seemed to have been doing so for years. Bart felt as if he was crashing some kind of exclusive boys' club. He had decided beforehand that he couldn't exactly say he was from On-Site Gas in Newington, Connecticut, and had concocted what he thought was an impressive-sounding name of a medical company for which he said he was the representative. Therefore he introduced himself as "Bart Gullong, vice president of Med-Equip." No one had any idea who Bart Gullong was.

Dacorta reviewed the protocol for the trial, which would be held in a week's time. "Seven hundred-odd pound pigs," Dacorta said, "will be anesthetized and cut in the femoral artery, a hundred percent lethal injury if left untreated." The injury model that Dacorta and his colleagues had created for the trial, he explained, was based on Jamie Smith's fatal wound at Mogadishu. Having been a medic for twenty years, Dacorta liked to base product tests on actual cases rather than theoretical constructs from the lab. Smith's injury was, for that purpose, ideal: it was well documented and set the ultimate standard for assessing a blood clotting product's capacity to save a soldier's life. Smith, of course, had died. As far as Dacorta was concerned, the goal of the trial was to find a product that would have saved him.

Immediately the doctors around the table began to aggressively critique Dacorta's protocol. Bart saw that there was something unflappable about Dacorta, who remained even-keeled during these exchanges. It became clear that each of the scientists was trying to manipulate the protocol to align with his own product's best features. Bart said nothing—as he of course had no idea what the best features of zeolite were. Finally, Dacorta asked Bart if he had any concerns about how the trial was going to be conducted. "No," Bart said. "To me, that's sort of like asking a solider how he wants to be wounded." An uncomfortable silence followed.

A week later, Bart was back in the hospital for the trial. He was introduced to a soft-spoken navy surgeon, Hasan Alam. On the operating table was a sedated pig. Bart did not have permission to videotape the proceedings, but he had brought his own camcorder from home anyway and recorded Dr. Alam using a scalpel to cut a six-inch incision deep into the swine's thigh. Bart very much doubted that the zeolite was going to work. But on the remote chance that it did, he realized that shooting this video was his one opportunity to create unassailable visual evidence of its effectiveness. He made sure to record the operation in one continuous shot, not wanting anyone to challenge his video later by saying he had manipulated zeolite's effects with editing techniques. As Alam made his incision, blood immediately spurted out as if from a faucet. It was astonishing how much blood gushed from the wound. Then Alam poured the zeolite into the pool of blood and waited. For a few seconds, nothing at all happened, and Bart's heart sank. *Maybe Frank was wrong all along.* That, of course, was possible with Frank: he was just otherworldly enough to allow himself to be deluded. But then Bart saw the blood begin to slow. At first the change was almost imperceptible, but then the flow of blood began to slow some more, and then some more, and after ten or fifteen seconds it clearly—undeniably now—became sluggish and heavy. A thrill ran through Bart. Bart was delighted by what he had just witnessed, but he didn't want to get his hopes up too high; after all, he had no idea how any of the competing products performed. And if Dr. Alam and his assistants were impressed, they didn't show anything. They worked in complete silence. As Bart was ushered out, he asked an attendant if any of the pigs, were they to perish, might be donated to a food pantry or something. The attendant laughed. "No," he said.

When Bart arrived at the office the next day, Frank said, "Well, how did it go?"

"Pretty well," Bart said, and showed him the tape.

"Looks good to me," Frank said. But he didn't appear to be especially excited. Certainly the visual evidence in Bart's video was promising, but they both knew there were many uncertainties involved in working with the military, especially in their position as outsiders. They shouldn't count on anything, they agreed. You never knew with the military where things might lead, or if they would lead anywhere at all. In fact, Bart pretty much put zeolite in the back of his mind and returned to selling oxygen generators.

But two weeks later, Bart's phone rang. It was Dr. Alam.

"Mr. Gullong?" the doctor said.

"Yes," Bart said.

"You have quite a product there, Mr. Gullong."

"Really?"

"Yours did by far the best of all the agents we tested. In fact, yours was the only one in which none of the pigs died."

"Really?" Bart said again, flabbergasted.

"Actually, I think you may have an historic product," Alam said at the end of the conversation.

Once he was off the phone, Bart ran to Frank, who was in his new, large, and almost entirely empty corner office. There was hardly any furniture in the room, and Frank hadn't put anything up on the walls or really bothered to decorate at all. As Bart relayed the news, Frank now smiled broadly. So he had been right about the "void spaces." But still Frank wasn't especially animated: after all, he'd already known that zeolite clotted blood. He had known this for seventeen years, going back to the time when he had first conducted his basement experiment. No, Frank seemed more satisfied than anything else, gratified to hear that the world had finally caught up to what he had known for decades.

But Bart was excited. In the moments after talking to Dr. Alam and Frank, Bart had a flash vision of what the next part of his life was going to look like. He saw it all in front of him. It was those words *historic product* that set him off. Bart suddenly realized, with a kind of fierce certainty, that as a result of meeting Frank, he had just walked into the opportunity of a lifetime. He had been looking all his life for a transformational product, one that would make a truly positive impact, and just maybe he had found one. But he was also scared. He knew he was going to be entering the world of the American military, which was among the largest and most opaque bureaucracies in existence. He knew that he and Frank would probably be considered rank amateurs.

Bart knew that in order to be a successful salesperson, you had to know your customer. From bitter experience he had learned that even an excellent product would fail without a customer who appreciated it. After his coaching career, Bart had developed a product in the early 1990s, a digital speedometer for rowing shells. He called it Speed Boss. It worked well, giving the coxswain the stroke rate and speed of the boat in real time. He had developed Speed Boss relatively quickly with a friend, but the engineering had been tricky;

it was hard to extrapolate a speed from the herky-jerky nature of a rowing shell in action on the water. He traveled to England to demonstrate his invention to a boating company, and to the Head of the Charles Regatta in Boston, where he showed the product's capabilities to all the leading coaches. Bart believed that with his innovation he was going to usher the old-fashioned sport of rowing into the digital, high-tech age and give those who bought Speed Boss a significant competitive advantage. But all the coaches, save for the MIT coach, were entirely disinterested. Five years later, Bart sold Speed Boss to a sports instrumentation company for $70,000, a not-inconsiderable sum but nothing like what he had hoped for. He realized later that he had misjudged his customer. Rowing coaches are a spartan bunch disinclined to use technology and interested in maintaining their singular power over their athletes. Speed Boss gave information only to the coxswain in the boat, not to the coach in the launch. Bart had learned that without a customer you had nothing. When it came to the zeolite invention, Bart feared that military officers and their egos were going to act just like the Ivy League crew coaches.

As he drove home that night to Sarah and Linda, all of it came crashing down on him. This product perhaps had the potential to save lives. It was also probably going to be his last shot at redemption. *I cannot afford to screw this up. Holy shit*, he thought to himself, *what the hell do I do now?*

PART TWO

THE WARS

Guerilla war is a kind of war waged by the few
but dependent on the support of many.
— Captain B. H. Liddell Hart, British
military historian

CHAPTER FOUR

The Rower

OVER THE NEXT few weeks, that phrase *historic product* continued to echo through Bart's mind. It simultaneously inspired and scared him. Of course, Bart didn't know Dr. Alam well—they had met at the trial only two weeks previously—but Bart was a quick study, and he could tell that the doctor was not one to dramatize or exaggerate matters.

Dr. Alam had received his medical degree in his native Pakistan and been chief resident in surgery at Washington Hospital Center affiliated with Georgetown University, and then a staff surgeon at the Uniformed Services University of the Health Sciences, the leading medical school for military doctors. He had been on duty on 9/11 when a plane flew into the Pentagon. Alam had been part of the team that cared for the victims. After the tragedy, like John Holcomb before him, he'd switched his career from a clinical one to one based in research. He decided he wanted to make an impact on a larger and more enduring scale, even though the new focus on research meant a significant reduction in pay for his young family. By the time of the zeolite trial, he had written forty papers and been awarded $1 million in grants from the navy and the National Institutes of Health to conduct studies on hemorrhagic shock. A few years previously, he had applied through Michael Given to the Office of Naval Research for a grant to study fluid resuscitation—that is, techniques to restore blood volume after trauma. But with war being waged in Afghanistan, he'd discussed with Dr. Given the idea of reallocating the grant to run a trial that would evaluate hemostatic agents. Stopping bleeding on the battle-field now seemed more urgent. Alam was shocked when Given reallocated the funds to address what he agreed was the more pressing priority.

Bart was also worried about the practical work involved in bringing the zeolite product to fruition. He knew that if zeolite was ever to be actually deployed by the marines and the navy in a war zone, complex preparatory work would be required, work that Bart knew very little about. For example, during their conversation, Alam had asked Bart if zeolite was FDA approved.

Bart was about to say: *Are you kidding? We just got it out of the barrel a month ago in Connecticut and put it in the microwave.* Instead he said, simply, "No."

Alam replied, in his cordial fashion, "Well, we will have to look into that. The FDA is not particularly within my scope of expertise. I will refer you to the navy program director, Lieutenant Commander Dacorta, for that question." Bart remembered Dacorta from the preliminary meeting before the trial. He had been impressed by Dacorta; Bart recalled how he hadn't been intimidated by the arrogance of some of the scientists and had treated Bart, an uncredentialed newcomer, as an equal, on the same footing as the doctors and biochemists from the other companies who had been working on their products in some cases for years.

Bart wondered, how does one even get FDA approval, particularly for a ground-up rock that has been used only in industrial machines and never once as a treatment for humans? Where would you even start? Certainly there would have to be testing and clinical trials, all of which he knew would be expensive and time consuming. Bart also knew that Frank had no interest in funding such research. Even though On-Site Gas was making good profits now, Frank retained his father's Depression-era attitudes about money and often feared that the business could go under at any time. The process, even if Bart and Frank could somehow pull it off with virtually no resources, would probably take five years, even a decade. Even Big Pharma needed years to bring a new drug to market. By then, Bart knew, the opportunity would be long gone, and no matter how estimable a physician-researcher he was, no one would care that Dr. Alam had once called zeolite a "historic product."

As literary and verbal as Bart could be—in college he had been an English major and had read all of Shakespeare, and *Moby-Dick* four times over—he often saw the world in pictures, even fables. In moments of stress, or at turning points in his life, an image or story would often appear in his mind. Later, when he looked back at a given period in his life, the image that he had assigned to that time would immediately come to him, allowing him instant access to his memories. His years in the Hamptons—most of his thirties and the entire decade of his forties—in which he had spent too much time in bars, despised himself for flipping houses and selling yachts to people who didn't care about sailing, and gone through many girlfriends and a marriage, were tied in his mind to Aesop's fable

"The Ant and the Grasshopper." In the story, a colony of ants and a grasshopper live in a field over a summer. While the grasshopper plays and makes music all summer, the ants toil away, storing food for the winter. As fall approaches, the grasshopper asks the ants for food. "Why haven't you stored anything away for the winter?" the ants ask. "I didn't have time to store up any food," whines the grasshopper. "I was so busy making music that before I knew it, the summer was gone." The ants turn away from the grasshopper in disgust, leaving him to starve. Over that entire decade, Bart had seen himself as the grasshopper, partying the summer away. But since he'd met Frank, he had become a hardworking ant.

But the most enduring self-image that Bart used to define his life—the entire arc of his life, or at least his life since he was thirteen—was that of a rower, a portrait of an oarsman out on a lake or river. As a coach on the US national women's team in 1974, when he was twenty-five years old, he had always told his athletes, "Rowing is not that hard of a sport. Technically, anyway. It doesn't require the incredible hand-eye coordination and dazzling skill of many sports. If you are a decent enough athlete, you can learn the basics of rowing pretty quickly. But in fact, rowing is the most difficult sport. Aerobically it punishes the body more than anything else. It is the most painful. And the key to success in rowing is that the team that can take the most pain usually wins."

Rowing surely had taught Bart tenacity, but it had also taught him pain: how to understand pain, how to manage it, how to endure it, and how to take on more of it than one's opponent. Even though he had left the sport twenty years before, he still considered his life as that of an oarsman. Ever since he'd received the telephone call from Dr. Alam, as he processed the implications of the news, Bart had seen himself at the starting line of a crew race.

Bart had always defined himself in relation to water, having spent much of his youth messing around in boats on Cornfield Point, a three-quarter-mile-long spit of beachfront in Old Saybrook, where his parents had a cottage. Most of the few good times he had with his father were on an outboard motorboat on Long Island Sound when Bart was a boy. When he was thirteen his father gave him a small fiberglass speedboat, and he spent hours alone careening around the sound, marveling in the freedom and possibilities of open water. That same year, he and a friend, on a mutual dare, broke into an empty community pool club during the winter. A neighbor heard the disturbance and called the police. Bart was brought home in the back of a police officer's cruiser. Bart's parents decided a change of scene was in order, and a few weeks later they gave him a book that described all the prep schools in New England. His mother said to Bart, "Pick one." Bart's selection was Tabor Academy in Marion, Massachusetts, at the mouth of Cape Cod. Tabor described itself as "the School by the Sea" and was known as a formal and traditional institution, renowned for its rowing and sailing prowess and marine science courses.

The next fall, Bart arrived at Tabor, a physically and sometimes socially awkward kid. He was tall and lanky, but not conventionally athletic, and couldn't throw a ball. He was an upper-middle-class boy in a school dominated by rich families that had gone to Tabor over generations. He was teased mercilessly. Sometime during his first semester, he was thrown by a group of classmates into the frigid waters of Buzzards Bay. A boy who was an onlooker to the scene said to Bart, "You're so goddamn weak." And then, as a sneering joke, the boy added, "Why don't you try crew? I am sure you'll be just great at it, you pussy."

The following day Bart tried out for the crew team. Tabor had been one of the first American prep schools to establish a rowing program, in 1909. In the 1930s Tabor had regularly rowed against colleges like Yale, Harvard, and MIT. For decades Tabor teams had competed at the world-famous regatta in Henley-on-Thames, England, and won a number of championships. It turned out that Bart had the right build for rowing: there was torque in his long limbs. There was also untapped rage in him, and he poured all of it into the oar. Having been around Long Island Sound his whole life—and the Tabor crews rowed not on lakes or rivers, but out on the bay—Bart understood winds and currents and the movement of water. He connected to the existential quality of the sport, which was about being simultaneously alone but also part of a team, and reveled in the difficult task of moving a large, ungainly piece of wood a mile in four minutes against the often uncooperative forces of nature. Quickly he picked up the mechanics and rhythms of rowing technique—how to "feather" one's oars and the art of following the stroke's lead. He grew to understand deeply the phys-ics of rowing—what conditions would produce the highest speed and which wouldn't—and found himself walking around campus thinking about optimal stroke rates. Over his first two years on the Tabor squad, Bart mainly rowed in the third boat of six, a considerable achievement given Tabor's prowess in the sport. The teasing by his classmates stopped.

In his senior year, he was catapulted to the second boat as the result of a single moment during a race. Bart's eight-man shell was competing against those of two high schools on Lake Quinsigamond in central Massachusetts. Tabor was leading but fell behind in an instant because the rower in the stroke position who set the pace "caught a crab"—that is, lost control of his oar when the blade got trapped in the water. The boat stopped dead. Out of frustration, Bart let out a guttural yell and heaved the shell forward with a single stroke filled with all the power he had within him.

It was as if he were purging himself of all the pain he held inside him—the abuse from his father, the teasing by his classmates, the constant assertions that he was not good enough. Because he was in the seventh seat directly behind the stroke position, that single action snapped the rest of the rowers back into rhythm. The shell surged ahead, and Tabor went on to win. The moment was caught on film by a coach recording the event. By the next practice Bart was elevated to the second boat and stayed there for the rest of his career. Years later, Bart would look back on this as one of the most significant events of his life. It wasn't about winning the race or getting promoted. It was that he learned, in that moment, what he was capable of. That single massive stroke was among the most profound things he had ever experienced, in its own way as profound as growing up with a depressed and angry father. He had learned that at his best he could will things to happen.

It would seem axiomatic that Bart, as a good student and a fine rower, would continue on to an elite New England liberal arts college. But in his senior year, Bart seemed to want to evade that path. In his application for Trinity College, a rowing powerhouse and his mother's alma mater, he wrote an essay entitled "The Death of the Liberal Arts." During the Harvard application process, he got into an argument with the interviewer. Late in the fall semester, at one of the many college fairs at Tabor, Bart spoke to the representative from Marietta College in southern Ohio, an established liberal arts college with a strong rowing tradition dating back to 1831. His interest in the school was piqued when the representative said that Marietta did not require an application essay. In fact, she said she would help him write his application. That sounded just right to Bart.

He arrived at Marietta College in the fall of 1966 and joined the crew team and a fraternity. Marietta was in a sleepy town in southern Ohio. If Bart had wanted to get away from New England elitist mores, he had succeeded. Only the Ohio River—where Bart rowed—separated Marietta from West Virginia and nearby Kentucky. Marietta seemed more part of the South than the North. He grew to love Marietta—if not the college itself then certainly his classmates. He found them interesting and bright people who had eschewed the more traditional institutions. There he grew his hair long and learned to question things. He gravitated away from crew and toward women, read deeply and widely in his English classes, and joined the anti–Vietnam War movement. He joined the hippie movement to the extent that he vowed in college that he was going to try to do something good for the world before he died—to leave not a material legacy behind him but rather a contribution to humanity that would last beyond his lifetime. But he also had other agendas. In the summer of 1969, he went to the Woodstock festival in upstate New York not so much for the music as for the opportunity to make money. He and a friend bought a carload of soda and food and sold it at a great profit at the festival. In his junior year, Bart worked on his fraternity brother Earle Maiman's campaign to be president of the student body. Once elected, Earle spoke out about the Vietnam War and what he saw as the hypocrisy of the faculty members who supported it. Six days later, Maiman was expelled. A campus revolt ensued. Much of the student body boycotted classes for two days, and one hundred students went on a hunger strike. Almost half of the student body, including Bart, joined a candlelit "funeral march" for free speech. At his graduation in the spring of 1970, Bart's father said that if his son protested the war by donning a peace sign on his mortarboard, he would not speak to him for a week. Bart wore the peace sign. His father, taking his wife and Bart's sister with him, left the ceremony before seeing Bart graduate and drove directly back to Connecticut.

In the summer of 1970, Bart lived at home in Connecticut, and in the fall he enrolled in a master's degree program in counseling at Central Connecticut State University. He thought he might want to pursue a career in education. As part of his degree, he did an internship at Simsbury High School, located in a rural but upscale suburb of Hartford. He would get up at four thirty in the morning, go to the high school, do his practicum, and then attend night classes, returning home at eleven at night. At least in this way he avoided his father. Bart was popular with his students at the high school, and one day he casually mentioned the idea of starting a rowing team. The students responded. In the winter of 1971, he lined up forty potential rowers and arranged for three shells to be loaned to him by Fred Emerson, a wealthy member of the US rowing Olympic committee and a well-known rowing benefactor in Connecticut. Emerson, who was in his fifties, lived in tony Old Lyme, adjacent to Old Saybrook, and Bart had borrowed single-person shells from him during high school summers to get some extra practice in. Bart started up the first crew team in Simsbury High School's history, and he immediately proved to be a relentless coach. In the winter, the team members lifted weights and ran. As soon as it was warm enough, they went to a lake in Massachusetts, where Bart taught them the sport. But before they took to the water for practice, Bart had them run five miles.

But their first season appeared to be over before it even started. Bart had recruited two girls to be coxswains for the boys' team. This was before the federal Title IX ruling that established equity across genders in publicly funded education. Simsbury's administrators heard there were girls on the team and closed the program before the first race. The *Hartford Courant* wrote a story about the cancellation of the team, and the piece was picked up by the Associated Press and went national. Bart and his athletes maneuvered to have the team operate as a private club, which allowed them to have girls as coxes. He raised funds by organizing submarine sandwich sales. In the first season of Simsbury rowing, Bart's team won two of the five state championships.

In the fall of 1971, there was an opening for the coach of both the men's and women's crew at Connecticut College in New London, a genteel and prestigious liberal arts college that had recently gone coed, accepting men for the first time. Emerson recommended Bart and arranged to pay his salary. Bart was an even more intense coach at Conn College than he had been at Simsbury. He conducted eleven practices a week at the borrowed Yale boathouse on the nearby Thames River. Bart wore a blazer and tie most days but sported a rakish moustache, and his hair was long over the collar. He wasn't much older, of course, than the students. "I am what I am," he told the student newspaper. "I'd rather go out drinking with the students than have tea with the faculty." In the fall of 1972, a record sixty students tried out for crew, equally divided between men and women. The student newspaper wrote that "the biggest thing that has hit Connecticut College since it [went coed] has been the appointment of Bart Gullong."

He proved a natural if at times bombastic marketer for the sport and inspired his athletes to work beyond expectations. At the start of each season, he would say, "In the future, you will forget courses you took, you will forget names of professors. You will forget names of your classmates. You will never forget every single stroke of every race." The students would laugh at him and then tell him later it was true. On February 1, 1973, Gullong audaciously sent an open letter to crew coaches in the Northeast, suggesting Conn College as the training center for women rowers preparing for the 1976 Olympics, where women rowers would compete for the first time. Bart's record by the end of the 1973 season was 20–6 for the women's varsity, second in the nation, and 9–7 for the men's. The campus paper ran an article about him: "Bart Gullong: Stroke of Genius."

By this time Bart had four women rowers who were at a national level. He received a call from Gus Constant, the well-known women's coach at Vesper Boat Club in Philadelphia, the nation's leading club, asking him to help coach the team competing for the 1974 national championship. Constant asked Bart to bring his four top rowers with him. That summer, Bart and his four rowers lived in a dangerous neighborhood in north Philly. It was one of the hottest summers on record, and there were sounds of gunfire at night. Bart and Constant worked the women hard on the Schuylkill River. At the end of the summer the Vesper 8 won the gold at the US women's championship by an impressive seven seconds over Radcliffe in a thousand-meter course in Lake Merritt, California. Half the team was comprised of Bart's recruits from Conn College. Later that year, Bart traveled with the Vesper team to Lucerne, Switzerland, to compete for the world championship. They finished sixth in the final for the runner-up teams, a huge disappointment. Still it had been a remarkable run in just a few years.

In the fall of 1974, the president of Connecticut College met with Gullong and effectively opened up the checkbook for him. He told Bart that he could become solely a full-time crew coach, giving up his additional job as director of the campus center, that his salary would be doubled, and that he would receive housing on Faculty Row. Bart was twenty-five years old. For someone who had devoted the last decade to crew, it was a dream come true. But strangely something shivered in Bart during the conversation. As the college president laid out his golden future—one that would no doubt have him coaching at the college for the next forty years, most likely winning national championships—something in him went cold. *It's great, sure, but would that be all there is?* He would grow old and die on the shores of the Thames River. Surely there could be more to his life legacy than that.

On January 30, 1975, the college newspaper ran a rather terse article, "Bart Gullong Leaves Conn," stating that as of February 1— two days later—Gullong was leaving campus. Citing personal reasons and "a job offer he couldn't refuse," Gullong was taking a new position as director of student affairs at Southampton College in Southampton, New York, on the lower fork of eastern Long Island.

At every level it was a strange move. He had just been offered what amounted to a lifetime tenure. Connecticut College had a long and worthy reputation, while Southampton College had been established only a decade earlier and would go on to cease operations as an independent institution in 2005. Most pointedly, Southampton didn't even have a rowing program. In leaving Conn College, he was leaving the sport behind entirely. In just a few years, Bart had grown sick of the parochialism and tradition-bound strictures of the established rowing world. Bart would spend only three indifferent years at Southampton before he resigned, starting a relatively short-lived video game company, and left the college world—and working for any kind of institution or company, for that matter—for good.

Bart's experience at Conn College and at Southampton presaged a pattern that would come to characterize his entire career: short bursts of brilliance that did not always sustain themselves. He was beginning to realize that his real interest was in starting a business more than operating one. As a true entrepreneur, he most liked to create things. In other words, he was more engaged in building the plane than flying it.

But now zeolite, if Dr. Alam was right, might give him a last shot at victory. He was beyond middle age now, and he only had so many chances left. When he felt overwhelmed by the anxiety and fear of trying to deliver on the potential of zeolite, Bart liked to think that he was now where he most liked to be—at the start of a race. That was where he was at his best.

———————

A few weeks after the blood clotting trial, Bart and Frank received the results of the investigation. The chart read as follows:

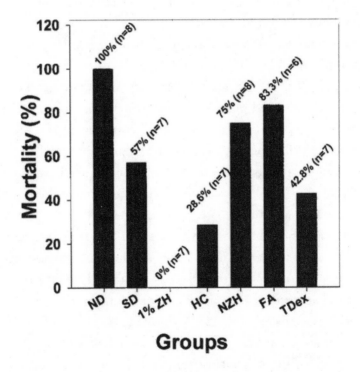

HC stands for HemCon. ZH is zeolite. SD stands for standard gauze, and ND for no dressing.

Bart studied the graph. He was momentarily thrown off by the fact that zeolite had the lowest bar—in fact, it had no bar at all. "But I thought we did well," Bart said.

"We did. That means no pigs died," Frank said, pointing to the word *Mortality* along the y-axis. "Zero mortality for us," he said triumphantly, a rare hint of pride in his voice.

Joe Dacorta, Tom Eagles, and Bart had a conference call a week later to review the results. The reality of what had transpired had begun to sink in for all of them: a mineral that none of them had ever heard of—that *nobody* had ever heard of—had bested every other agent in the trial. Dacorta couldn't help but ask Eagles, "Why did you even let these guys in on the trial? You didn't even really know them all that well."

"I don't know," Eagles said. "I just had a good feeling about them. And I liked Bart. He made me laugh."

Regarding FDA approval, Dacorta explained that zeolite, as an inert substance, could possibly be construed as a "medical device" rather than a drug. This, he explained, could be a game changer. The threshold for the approval of medical devices was far lower: you had to prove efficacy—which it could be argued that Alam and Dacorta already had—but you didn't have to conduct the expensive and years-long randomized clinical trials required for pharmaceutical products. Second, Dacorta said, given that the country was at war, it could be argued that the use of zeolite was "mission critical" to national security. But that, Eagles explained, would require a letter from at least a four-star general or admiral.

"And how would I do that?" Bart asked.

"Let me see what I can do," Eagles said. "I know Peter Pace, the commander of the Marine Corps, well. I helped him survive the Vietnam War when I was a medic. In fact I pulled him out of a ditch one time."

A week afterward, Bart was in his office in Connecticut when the fax machine began to stir. The digital register on the machine said a document was being sent from Eagles's office in Quantico. Out came a document with a letterhead reading "Commandant, United States Marine Corps, The Pentagon." The letter was brief but emphatic: it said that Frank Hursey's discovery of zeolite as a blood clotting agent was "mission critical" to the war on terror. It was signed by General Peter Pace, commander of the Marine Corps.

For once, Bart was unable to speak. He took a moment to collect himself before calling Eagles.

"I just got this letter from General Pace," Bart said.

"Yeah, I know. Hell, it only took me half a day to get his signature right!" Eagles said.

Bart couldn't believe that Eagles had had the temerity to do such a thing. But in time he learned this was just another example of Eagles's sense of humor. Dacorta said that Eagles had spoken to the general, who had taken Eagles's word that this was a lifesaving product, and signed the letter.

With things moving forward so quickly, Bart and Frank realized that they needed to give the product an actual name. Bart went into his office, closed the door, and took out a yellow legal pad. He jotted down ideas for an hour. A good product name, Bart knew from sales experience, met three criteria: it had to be short, it had to be memorable, and it had to describe what the thing actually did. The choice of the right name was critical. A good product could be killed by a bad name.

He wrote in loopy, sloppy handwriting the following candidates: *Fastclot, Instaclot, Broadcloth, Stopquick, Bloodstop*. None of them seemed quite right. *Bloodstop* was perhaps the most compelling and accurate, but it also seemed a little unseemly—too graphic. He then broke the parts of the words up—*fast* and *clot* and *quick* and *insta*—and re-arranged them, as if he were playing a word game. He tried them in different combinations, arranging them in all the orders he could think of. One declared itself on the page immediately. *QuickClot.* QuickClot! Or maybe—taking out the *c* to make it even shorter—QuikClot. And there it was. Memorable, brief, saying in only eight letters what the product actually did. There was a parallel between the two short words, and an appealing sharpness to the *k* sounds. QuikClot. That was it! An hour had passed since he'd started.

He went to find Frank.

"QuikClot," Bart said. "What do you think?"

"I like it," Frank said.

And then they realized that if they were going to have a product, they would have to have a separate company—not On-Site Gas Systems—to produce it. And if they were going to have a separate company, it would need a name beyond Med-Equip, the name Bart had used at the trial. Bart once again went to his office and took out his yellow legal pad. The name would have to differentiate itself from On-Site Gas and announce decisively that it was a medical company, not a technology company. Frank had suggested they use the word *medical,* or some variation of it, in the title. And why not feature a letter like *x* or *y* or *z,* the way so many drug and medical companies did, to convey a feeling of sharpness or exactitude? Bart wrote down the letters. Z immediately popped out. Of course, it would have to be *z,* standing for *zeolite.* The name came to him within five minutes. He wrote it down in his large handwriting: "Z-MEDICA."

He walked back to Frank's office. "What do you think?" Bart said.

"I like that too," Frank said.

On a handshake, Frank made Bart CEO of the new company.

Bart immediately got down to the work of product design and

production. There were many details to figure out: the kind of packaging the military required, the directions to be printed on the product, how and where the QuikClot package would be placed in soldiers' first-aid kits. He went to a conference on industrial packaging in Chicago and came away realizing that a QuikClot package would have to look suitably rugged and feature military camouflage colors. It would need to have a simple, utilitarian, but somehow urgent look. He learned the vicissitudes of vacuum packaging at another conference. Working with Eagles and Dacorta, Bart settled on how much a packet should contain—a hundred grams, or 3.5 ounces of zeolite, plenty of material to treat a massive wound. They priced the packet at twelve dollars—remarkably inexpensive, but then again, zeolite was inexpensive.

The first packages of QuikClot were in a camel-yellow camo-style color, the lettering in simple black blocks. On the package was written:

QuikClot
Adsorbent Hemostatic Agent Temporary Traumatic Wound Treatment
To Stop Moderate-to-Severe Bleeding
By Promoting Rapid Coagulation
For External/Emergency Use

Meanwhile, Dacorta guided Frank and Bart through the testing of QuikClot against further safety standards—to prove, for example, that it wasn't corrosive to the touch—at an independent lab. The testing would cost $2,300. Frank recoiled at the expense when Bart brought it up. "We can't afford that! If the tests fail, who's going to pay for it? Me?" he said.

"No, Frank, we'll split it," Bart responded. "Whether the product passes the safety test or not, I will pay for half." The offer seemed to make a dramatic impression on Frank and proved to be a turning point in their relationship. It showed Frank that Bart was as invested as he, perhaps even more so, in the success of the project.

With everything now moving quickly, Bart asked Frank to produce the original patent for zeolite he had long talked about, which Frank said he had filed away at home in West Hartford.

"Sure, I will get it tonight," Frank said.

The next morning, a ghostly-looking Frank appeared in the office and said, "I am so sorry. I found the papers last night. The patent expired years ago. Apparently I didn't pay the renewal fees."

Bart couldn't believe it. *We're gonna fuck this up now? Or actually: Frank is going to fuck this up now?* He felt like slamming Frank's entire face into his desk. But outwardly he kept calm. Frank was devastated and it would be cruel to make him feel worse. But it was deeply discouraging—this could set them back years.

Bart contacted the best patent attorney in Hartford to investigate what exactly had happened and what could be done. The attorney came back with even worse news. He not only confirmed that Frank's patent had long since expired but also informed Bart that a scientist in 1999 had submitted a patent, approved in 2000, that effectively co-opted Frank's original patent. It was ten pages long, compared to the little more than a page Frank had written for his submission. The ten pages were elegantly written, meticulously researched, and clearly the work of an accomplished scientist. But the true genius of the patent lay in how broad it was. It was not for a particular invention but rather for a general method to create hemostasis—that is, to stop bleeding. The scientist had created a method of facilitating clotting through the introduction into a wound of a purified potato-based powder that absorbed water in blood. But beyond that, the scientist had created an intellectual property that covered a *method* of stopping bleeding—that is, adding something that sponged up the water in blood, leaving the clotting factors, which had been Frank's original insight. The scientist's patent worked as a kind of umbrella patent that now covered the way zeolite worked too. And this meant, Bart realized with horror, that Frank and he were now *working in violation of their own idea.* The scientist had them cornered.

"Who the fuck is this guy," Bart asked the patent attorney, "and what's his product and company?"

The attorney said the company's name, which sounded familiar to Bart. The company had been represented at the trial, Bart realized. It had not done that well. A number of the pigs had died.

Bart picked up the phone and called the company. He played the naive newcomer to the field. He tried to sound like an amateur, a scientific nobody. "Look, we might have a potential stalemate," Bart told the scientist. "But we also have some common ground and some common interests. Would you be up for me flying out to see you to discuss a few things with you?" To his surprise the scientist said yes.

One way or the other, Bart had dealt with academics his whole life. He knew they liked to be flattered. Bart flew across the country, and once having arrived at the scientist's office, he began the meeting by saying, "You guys did an amazing job. You have the product that will do the job. You are the ones who have the more doable project. We're just new to this. And remember, both of us are really just doing first aid here, nothing medical, an area that is totally devalued in medicine. This is not really that important to the military. They are after bigger things."

The scientist appeared weirdly receptive to this argument. He seemed to agree that his product was intriguing but not ultimately sophisticated science.

"So," Bart said, "we are walking the same street. But the street is very big, and we are doing something quite different. How about we write something up that we get to do our own thing, and you do your thing? An agreement. It will say we won't sue you, and you won't sue us. Sound fair?"

The scientist nodded.

Still, Bart left the meeting unclear if he had actually succeeded. But back in Connecticut, he wrote a letter for the company to sign, allowing Z-Medica to proceed with its zeolite invention unimpeded. He overnighted it, with return express mail posted. The signed and fully executed letter came back to Bart in a couple of days. Once again Bart went to Frank's office to let him know the astonishing news. Frank smiled and said, "You did good, Bart," perhaps not realizing the full magnitude of what Bart had pulled off.

The way forward now clear, Tom Eagles and Joe Dacorta then referred Bart to the FDA officer in charge of hemostatic products, Dr. David Krause, who also turned out to be a reservist marine. It seemed to be a good omen. On May 24, 2003, a remarkable two months after the trial, QuikClot was approved by the FDA.

The process of readying the product for deployment proceeded quickly. By August, Dacorta made his first order of three thousand packets of QuikClot at about ten dollars each. That was followed by seven much larger orders. But those in army medicine, led by John Holcomb, continued to show no interest in QuikClot. The army announced it was formally electing to go with HemCon as its blood clotting agent, leaving the marines and navy to go with QuikClot. It was a classic case of interservice rivalry—in this case the army versus the marines and the navy—which was something the military had long prided itself on.

But there was controversy from the beginning. The army selected HemCon even though it was far more expensive—at seventy-nine dollars a bandage—than QuikClot and there were emerging doubts about its practicality and effectiveness. Nonetheless, HemCon had received expedited approval from the FDA in November 2002, the second-fastest approval in the administration's history. And even the skeptics agreed that the concept behind the bandage, and the process of producing it, amounted to a daring scientific and logistical feat. It involved buying shrimp shells in bulk from Iceland—and later from Hawaii after the Department of Defense allocated $4.5 million of procurements—and then boiling the shells in lye or sodium hydroxide to extract the chitosan, which was mixed with vinegar so it could be formed into a bandage. By contrast, QuikClot was a ground mineral that you simply dried up and poured into a wound.

Despite the brewing conflict between the two products, within a remarkable six months of the Alam trial, QuikClot was issued in the first-aid kits of navy corpsmen and marines in Iraq. The leading medical officer for the Marine Corps, Rear Admiral Robert Hufstader, requested roughly eighty thousand bags, which allowed QuikClot to be supplied for every marine going into combat. Dacorta and Eagles told Bart that the pace of development was unprecedented. Even the marines, known for their nimbleness and flexibility, never ever worked this fast, they said.

Bart and Frank simply couldn't believe it. *QuikClot is going to war!* Even Dacorta and Eagles and Alam did not fully comprehend it. It seemed a miracle, as much of one as the product itself.

But the celebrations were relatively short lived. Little did Bart and Frank know that that phrase—*QuikClot is going to war!*—would soon take on an ominous double meaning.

CHAPTER FIVE

The Wound-Dresser

DURING DR. ALAM'S trial of zeolite, Lieutenant Commander Joseph Dacorta of the navy had visited the operating room where the surgeries took place, but only briefly. His role was to design and organize the trial, not to conduct it. Dr. Alam had tested zeolite on seven pigs altogether, and Dacorta had been present for only two of the procedures. When Dacorta saw that zeolite dramatically halted the bleeding of the first pig, he was surprised and even mildly enthused. *That is impressive, but it's just one data point.* When the zeolite performed just as well on a second pig, he thought, *That is impressive too, but then again, it is just a second data point. Let's await the final results.* After all, Dacorta knew nothing about zeolite or the people behind it. He hadn't even heard of the product until a week earlier, when, somewhat reluctantly, he had allowed it to be entered into the trial as a personal favor to Eagles. It was highly unorthodox to add a candidate at the last minute.

At the time of the trial, Dacorta, in his early fifties, had been a navy medic and medical officer for twenty-five years. During that time he had witnessed many things that, while initially encouraging, ended up failing. He had spent almost three decades learning how important it was to distrust anything that looked too good to be true. He had also witnessed the American military, of which he was a devoted and faithful member, repeatedly fall short on the promises that it had made to its soldiers. And so when he saw two promising applications of zeolite, he was intrigued, but ultimately unmoved. He had made a career out of being skeptical.

Dacorta had always been something of an iconoclast in the military. Growing up as the oldest of six siblings in suburban Long Island, he'd spent a lot of his childhood sailing, sometimes alone, on the sound, just as Bart had. Starting in his early teens, he demonstrated a remarkable capacity to seek out and fully immerse himself in subjects that interested him, many somewhat obscure and scientific in nature, and all of them having very little to do with his schoolwork. He became intrigued by the ghostly remnants of the once-active farming community on Long Island and took up the study of local horticulture. Most of the topics he pursued, however, pertained to medicine. His father was a medical doctor, originally a general practitioner, who had retrained to become a community psychiatrist during the field's infancy. Dr. Dacorta worked at the state psychiatric facility with seriously and persistently mentally ill patients. Joe's mother was a nurse. She was also a devout Catholic and always involved in some kind of good work or other, such as coordinating donations for famine relief in Africa or running a bake sale for the elementary school. The bathroom reading in the Dacorta household was the *New England Journal of Medicine* and *JAMA*. Joe pored over a column at the back of each issue of *JAMA* edited by Morris Fishbein, which chronicled unusual case studies or episodes in the history of medicine. Fishbein took particular glee in exposing cases of medical quackery. Joe looked forward to reading

Fishbein's column the way his friends anticipated the arrival of *Sports Illustrated* or *Mad* magazine.

When Dacorta was in high school, his father sometimes brought him to the state hospitals and group homes where he worked, introducing him to his patients, who had typically been diagnosed with schizophrenia or bipolar disorder. Joe loved these encounters. He found talking to the patients fascinating, and he also appreciated seeing how his father worked with them, without bias or judgment. Mainly Dr. Dacorta just listened, and then on the drive home he would talk to his son with genuine interest about what Joe had observed during the encounters. These were somewhat rare moments of bonding between the two—Dr. Dacorta was usually distracted with work and, at times, aloof at home. The Dacortas lived very near the world-famous Cold Spring Harbor Laboratory, led by James Watson, who'd codiscovered the double helix structure of DNA. Joe's father was the on-call physician for the laboratory in the event of after-hours emergencies. Often the family would host a visiting international scholar for a week or so, and the talk around the dinner table, which might go on for hours, would be about the ethics of emerging DNA technology or the latest developments in neuroscience. Joe received the equivalent of a college education in medical issues before he finished high school.

Dr. Dacorta was also a World War II veteran. He had been a foot soldier in General George Patton's Seventh US Army division as it went from Africa north through Italy to Sicily. Joe noticed how guarded his father was about his war experiences; in fact, for all his openness about scientific matters, Dr. Dacorta never spoke of his enlistment and was quick to switch off the television if a war movie came on. Joe found this discrepancy in his father—the contrast between his intellectual expansiveness and his emotional restriction—both intriguing and frustrating. As he grew older and entered his teens, Joe developed a subinterest in the history of military medicine. Joe attended Walt Whitman High School on Long Island, where reading the poet was required. Most students laughed the assignments off, but Joe became haunted by Whitman. He was enamored with one poem in particular, "The Wound-Dresser," and it stuck with him from the first time he read it:

> *...Bearing the bandages, water and sponge,*
> *Straight and swift to my wounded I go,*
> *Where they lie on the ground after the battle brought in,*
> *Where their priceless blood reddens the grass, the ground,*
> *Or to the rows of the hospital tent, or under the roof'd hospital,*
> *...*
> *I onward go, I stop,*
> *With hinged knees and steady hand to dress wounds,*
> *I am firm with each, the pangs are sharp yet unavoidable,*
> *One turns to me his appealing eyes—poor boy! I never knew you,*
> *Yet I think I could not refuse this moment to die for you, if that would save you.*

After high school, Dacorta went to a small Jesuit college in upstate New York, where he read widely from the Western canon. He was particularly drawn to the empirical tradition of Thomas Aquinas, who argued that all concepts are derived from experience, or, as he wrote, that there is "nothing in the intellect which was not previously in the senses." Aquinas had stated what would become the predominant theme of Joe's later life and career: you should trust only what you can see and feel and hear right in front of you.

After college he joined the Peace Corps, spending two years in Jamaica, where he taught Rastafarians how to grow beans. "That was perhaps not the best idea ever," he said later. "They were more interested in another crop." He returned to the United States hoping to obtain a position in the Environmental Protection Agency or the Department of Agriculture, but it was the middle of the Carter-era recession, and the government wasn't hiring. Somewhat on a whim, in 1980 Dacorta joined the navy, where he was trained as a medic.

His higher-ups seemed to recognize the range and depth of his skills quickly. Joe began a peripatetic military career, pulled constantly into special projects and covert missions all over the world. In 1986 and 1987, he was in Guam and Palau, where he helped create medical protocols for the Pacific naval fleet. In 1991—two years before the Black Hawk Down incident—he was in Mogadishu helping American diplomats evacuate the US embassy after it was attacked. In 1994 he participated in the NATO humanitarian response to the genocide in Rwanda. In Bosnia and Herzegovina he was part of Operation Deny Flight, a NATO operation that enforced the UN resolution to establish a no-fly zone over those countries, and he supported the rescue of an air force pilot who had been shot down. He was in Ukraine delivering surplus medical equipment in 1995 and in Egypt helping to rescue passengers after a ferryboat went down in the Red Sea the following year. His typical role in these incidents was to assess and build medical capacity and infrastructure and on occasion to tend to the wounded. Like his father, he never spoke to anyone in any detail about his experiences in combat. As his military career wore on, Joe found that the true warriors never much spoke about their experiences. If pressed, he would say only, "Combat is the most irrational thing that humans do. It is kind of hard to put into words." Asked to detail the honors he'd received, he would simply say he was combat decorated. But when he returned home after a mission, the nightmares would start. They were always the same, or very similar—he was trapped somewhere, in a cave or the locked cabin of a truck. He was suffocating, couldn't move, and couldn't escape.

Dacorta was an inveterate wanderer. As far as the US Marines and navy were concerned, Dacorta was "our man in Mogadishu," then "our man in Rwanda," then "our man in Bosnia," and so on. There was an air of mystery as to why he was so frequently picked for such assignments. Of course, every career navy officer's number came up for such operations occasionally, but Dacorta's number seemed to come up all the time. When asked about this, he would scoff, "Well, clearly, they think I am the most expendable." But the main reason was that Dacorta would simply never say no to a request. Refusing, he felt, would violate his responsibility to his fellow sailors and soldiers. Besides, the missions, mainly, appealed to him. There was something inherently restless about him, and being asked to roam the world, sometimes on a few days'—or a few hours'—notice, was exciting, even intoxicating. Also, he was good at his work. He was calm under pressure, able to perform while in danger, unfazed by sleeplessness and long days, and he loved getting on a plane or helicopter or tank or boat. The more remote or unusual the place, the better. He was deeply interested in other cultures, and, like his father, a nonjudgmental student of other people, and he was particularly comfortable around people in distress. One of his favorite jobs had been visiting hospitals all over Africa to test EKG machines and other cardiological equipment and then filing an elaborate report of his findings. He was the ultimate combination of cultural anthropologist and pragmatic field-tester.

In his early thirties, Dacorta was given a yearlong fellowship in medicine, science, and technology at Virginia Tech. There he devoured philosophy and philosophy of science, and, unlike when he'd first read Thomas Aquinas in college, he now had a decade of experience tending to human suffering in all the corners of the world to bring to his studies. He experienced a rush of recognition and excitement when he read a passage that Descartes wrote in *Meditations on First Philosophy* in 1641:

> Several years have now elapsed since I first became aware that I had accepted, even from my youth, many false opinions for true, and that consequently what I afterward based on such principles was highly doubtful; and from that time I was convinced of the necessity of undertaking once in my life to rid myself of all the opinions I had adopted, and of commencing anew the work of building from the foundation.

In another piece of writing, Descartes summed up the entire philosophy of skepticism with the line *"Dubium sapientiae initium"* or "Doubt is the origin of wisdom."

Over the course of his career, Dacorta had learned to love and embrace doubt. He was proud of his service, but time and again he found that the American military in its certitude and arrogance failed to understand or even take into account local conditions and cultures, imposing its own theories and ideas without listening to what was really needed by the end user, whether that user was soldiers or victims of genocide in Rwanda. During the Gulf War, Dacorta was a detachment commander for a field surgical hospital preparing for an amphibious landing. He found that the Department of Defense had failed to modernize field training and equipment, even for basic items. He grew furious that the American military, with all its resources—with a budget that was at least triple that of any other country's armed forces, on par with the *entire* GNP of some major countries, like Switzerland—couldn't protect its soldiers. He saw firsthand that the forces behind that supply chain were often deeply inefficient. He came back from the Gulf War, as he put it, "wanting to kill the people in charge."

During the fellowship year, Dacorta also became immersed in the work of the twentieth-century Austrian philosopher of science Karl Popper, whose ideas had revolutionized the scientific method. Before Popper, scientific theories were generally tested through an ongoing process of verification. One developed a prediction, based on a theory, of what could occur under certain conditions. If the prediction was right, and the results repeated multiple times, the theory was verified and eventually became accepted as fact. Popper suggested the opposite should be the case. He believed that theories could be tested only if they could be falsified. Once they were falsified, they could then be tossed aside. In other words, one could prove only by disproving. Popper's famous example was the theory that all swans are white. He argued that no number of sightings of white swans would ever be enough to fully prove the theory, but the observation of a single black swan could falsify it. Popper saw the process of falsification as Darwinian: science evolves through natural selection, as theories gradually become extinct when they are disproven. Popper's version of the scientific method involved a whittling away of untruths until one is left not with the full truth, but with the best truth available under the circumstances. "The game of science is, in principle, without end," he wrote. "He who decides one day that scientific statements do not call for any further test, and that they can be regarded as finally verified, retires from the game."

In the years immediately before the Iraq War, starting in the mid-1990s, Dacorta transitioned out of the wandering part of his career and became jointly assigned to the Office of Naval Research and the Marine Corps Warfighting Laboratory in Quantico, where he worked for the mild-mannered Dr. Michael Given and Tom Eagles. By this point he was married and had two young daughters, and he wanted to see them grow up in suburban Virginia as a semi-normal parent. Dacorta felt immediately at home at the Office of Naval Research and at the Warfighting Lab. Both institutions were small, flexible, and remarkably unbureaucratic, which made for a dramatic contrast with Dacorta's experiences with army medicine. The organizational model for medical research within the navy and marines was entirely different from that of the army. The Office of Naval Research had minimal staff and facilities—90 percent of its funding went to external (that is, nonmilitary) scientists and experts. As Dr. Given put it, "We were facilitators. Our job was to take our funds and find the best people in the country to do their work and let them work independently. I set the goals and the parameters, but we trusted their autonomy and expertise." The Institute of Surgical Research took the opposite approach, conducting almost all of its work internally with the hundreds of doctors and research scientists in its massive facility in San Antonio. The navy and marines' budget for basic and early research was just a fraction of that of the army—less than 10 percent—but Dacorta took pride in the fact that even with far less support, he believed the navy and marines were at least as productive.

Michael Given valued the opportunity to work with Dacorta, finding his knowledge of medicine "encyclopedic." "It was like Joe could recall the outcome of every study he'd ever read," he says. "It was uncanny. But he was also practical. He knew that what might work in the lab might not work in the field, and he knew the world of military budgets, which had to prioritize multiple demands, many of them urgent, and simply couldn't support everything. Also, he could talk to anybody, whether it was a seventy-year-old scientist or a twenty-year-old marine." Dacorta met with Given weekly, but most of his days were spent in the Warfighting Laboratory, which despite its intimidating name was based in a modest, smallish house on the Quantico campus. Dacorta and Eagles bonded around their shared goal, born of their long personal histories of combat: to get the common soldier, sailor, or marine the medical equipment he needed to survive. Eagles was almost twenty years Dacorta's senior, but they complemented each other well. Eagles was affable where Dacorta was aloof; Eagles was intuitive where Dacorta was analytical; Eagles was the face of the department, while Dacorta mainly stayed behind the scenes, designing studies and reviewing data.

Dacorta knew that the methodology he would use to accomplish his goal of getting the best and most lifesaving equipment to soldiers needed to come straight out of Popper. Which is to say that as he evaluated new products or technologies, he would seek to falsify the claims made about them. He would remove the products that failed to deliver, no matter his personal feelings about them or the people who made them, and be left with the last product standing. Dacorta felt a sacred obligation to follow the evidence and only the evidence, and increasingly he had begun to chafe at John Holcomb and his evangelical fervor about the army's latest project or adoption. Dacorta knew all about the hype and then dismal failure of the army and Red Cross fibrin bandage. He recoiled whenever Holcomb used a word like *amazing* to describe something clinical or medical. Inwardly he would think, *You can't test "amazing." That's not objective. It is not even a word that belongs in science!*

Recently Dacorta had gotten annoyed by Holcomb's fervor about HemCon. Dacorta and Holcomb had known each other for ten years, seeing one another at the semiannual military trauma medicine conferences sponsored by the service branches. Often the conferences were held at a beachfront hotel in St. Petersburg, Florida, and representatives from private industry could also participate in some of the proceedings. Dacorta and Holcomb, or his army medicine team, would report on their work and research. Early on, Dacorta's relationship with Holcomb had been cordial, even collegial, but in recent years Holcomb had taken to pestering Dacorta about HemCon, trying to get him to buy quantities of it for the navy and marines. But Dacorta had tested HemCon before the trial and found it completely impractical. It wouldn't fit onto a wound unless the wound just happened to be the exact same shape as the bandage. How was that going to work in the real world? "I just don't get it, John," Dacorta told Holcomb. "How exactly is this supposed to work on the battlefield?"

In fact, Eagles and Dacorta had both grown to dislike almost everything about the army. They both shared a belief that the army had too much money, too much faith, and not enough proof for much of what it did. They also shared an affiliation with, and an affection for, the Marine Corps and its traditions, which they found to be the best part of American military culture. While Eagles and Dacorta were both naval personnel, in the curious arrangement through which the marines borrowed naval medical personnel, they worked almost exclusively in support of marines. They identified with the underdog, scrappy mentality of the marines and its ideology of doing more with less. At the Warfighting Laboratory, they enjoyed a minimum of bureaucratic interference and a large amount of freedom to make their own decisions. Perhaps for the first time in their careers, they felt liberated to use their now-extensive experience to find the best solutions to save soldiers' lives.

The mission of the US Marine Corps stems from its motto: *Semper Fidelis*, "always faithful." At its best, the fealty among marines, which is "to our Nation, the Corps, and to each other" is "not blind faith" but rather "a faith guided by our values." In this the marines seemed to Dacorta and Eagles to differ from the uglier aspects of the army, which could be monolithic, extraordinarily bureaucratic, and invested primarily in maintaining the army's dominance over other military branches. At its worst the army construed itself as bigger than the very nation—and indeed the army had been established before the creation of the Union. The marines had always been on the outside. Their branch had been formed during the American Revolution, and there had been from the beginning confusion about their role. Writing in the winter of 1776, Commander George Washington of the Continental Army asked one of his colonels whether the marines "resolved to act upon Land or meant to confine their Services to the Water only." The marines had constantly been under the threat of extinction throughout their history. The corps played a crucial role in Washington's raid on Trenton, but as soon as the war was over, both the Continental Navy and the marines were eliminated—only to be reestablished in 1798. More than a century later, the marines played a pivotal role during World War II, particularly in the Pacific. The corps grew from fifteen thousand regular duty personnel in 1940 to an astonishing 485,000 in 1945. But despite the marines' iconic success at, to pick only two examples, Iwo Jima and Okinawa—now forever part of national lore—the army attempted to disband the corps right after the war and divide it up between the army and the navy. Secretary of Defense Louis Johnson stated, "The navy is on its way out. There's no reason for having a navy and a Marine Corps. . . . We'll never have any more amphibious operations. That does away with the Marine Corps." President Harry Truman, who carried a hatred of the marines dating from his time in the army in World War I, wrote in a 1950 letter, "The Marine Corps is the navy's police force and as long as I am President, that is what it will remain. They have a propaganda machine that is almost equal to Stalin's." The Marine Corps survived only by virtue of congressional action in 1952.

But to Dacorta this checkered history was liberating. The marines had to be nimble in order to survive. There simply wasn't money to support an unwieldy bureaucracy. Indeed, at the beginning of the Iraq War, the army had nearly three times as many personnel as the marines and a budget four times as big. But to Dacorta this simply meant it was easier to get things done. As he was fond of saying, "When faced with an obstacle, a marine will either go around it, go through it, or simply remove it. Either way, there can be no whining."

The first project that Eagles and Dacorta undertook, largely led by Eagles, was the redesign of the individual first-aid kit (IFAK) carried by every soldier. The second project, led by Dacorta, was the creation of the Forward Resuscitative Surgical System, or FRSS—the portable operating room on the battlefield—which led to On-Site Gas being awarded the POGS contract. Dacorta viewed the FRSS as the necessary response to the changing nature of the battlefield. One of the many problems he had encountered during the Gulf War was that on the new battlefield, which was asymmetrical and moved fast, tanks and fighting vehicles outpaced medical battalions. The distance between the combat zone and the hospital could be 350 miles, and medical care was not readily available when soldiers were wounded. Dacorta saw a need for a surgical capability that was light enough to be carried in one medium logistics vehicle or aircraft, could be assembled in an hour, and was equipped to perform basic surgeries. He was put in charge of establishing the minimum essential requirements of the FRSS system, which included generators, operating tables, portable ventilators, and medical monitors of all kinds. In refining the oxygen generators for the system, Dacorta worked with Frank and Bart, and from the beginning, Bart and Dacorta worked easily together. They shared a dry sense of humor, and as scientifically astute as they both were, they were also literary and even philosophical types stranded in the field of technology. They both lived in a world inhabited by ideas and stories, not by organizational hierarchies and politics. Spurred by Eagles's credibility, Dacorta's expertise, and Bart's passion, the process of readying the product for deployment proceeded quickly. Dacorta's vision for the FRSS proved remarkably prescient. In just the first few months of the war in Iraq, 149 procedures were performed by the FRSS teams. Eight of those patients would have died if not for FRSS intervention.

And so when it came to the blood clotting trial, Joe Dacorta had the license to make the best decision based on the data, politics be damned. He also knew from personal experience how crucial that decision was going to be—that lives, potentially hundreds of them, were going to hang in the balance. The choice could either kill people or save them. Once the results were in, Dr. Alam and Dacorta sent them to all the companies represented. Using Popper's methodology, Dacorta had dismissed four of the products tested. These products were:

HemCon, from an Oregon company, with which 2 of the 7 pigs died
TraumaDex, from a Minnesota company, with which 3 of 7 pigs died
Rapid Deployment Hemostat, from a Massachusetts company, with which 4 of 6 pigs died
Fast Act Bovine Clotting factor, from a Tennessee company, with which 5 of 6 pigs died

Notably, some of the products had fared worse than standard gauze; with the application of gauze, only three of seven pigs had died.

Dacorta found it particularly difficult to break the disappointing news to the makers of the Rapid Deployment Hemostat bandage, a company called Marine Polymer Technologies. He and his colleagues at the Office of Naval Research had been working with that company for three years, commissioning and funding the bandage's development. Altogether, the staff at Marine Polymer had put almost ten years of work into the bandage, which, like HemCon, also used chitosan, although Marine Polymer's was derived from sea algae. But to Dacorta, of course, results were results, and the Marine Polymer bandage had failed in this trial, although the company later developed a successful hemostatic patch used widely in dialysis clinics.

However, Dacorta did not at all mind informing the HemCon company that its bandage had failed to perform well. In fact, on the day that HemCon was tested at the trial the bandage had done so poorly that out of professional courtesy Dacorta called a retired army colonel and doctor who had gone on to work for HemCon, and invited him to view the remaining applications of the bandage. The retired colonel seemed aggravated when Dacorta told him of the disappointing results and said that Alam must not be applying the bandage correctly. The colonel flew to Bethesda and observed the end of the trial. Dacorta recalled that the colonel, in person, had nothing substantive to suggest about how to better apply the bandage. Dacorta remembers seeing him turn a ghostly white as it continued to fail.

All that remained was for Dacorta to inform the representative of the only company whose claims for its product had not been falsified: Bart Gullong of the mysterious Med-Equip company, the man and company that no one at the trial had ever heard of. Dacorta couldn't help but take some glee in the result. It appealed to his absurdist sense of humor. Here a number of biotech companies led by accomplished scientists had been working for years on a clotting agent, investing collectively, by Dacorta's guess, hundreds of millions of dollars, and at the very last minute, two unknown and eccentric guys from Connecticut who had no medical or military training had found something that worked better than all of the other products put together. Dacorta chuckled as he picked up the phone.

But Dacorta told Bart and Frank that the real work lay ahead of them. Of the thousands of medical technologies the military had developed, only a handful had ever made it to the battlefield. Dacorta knew that the road would be particularly steep for Bart and Frank, who would be perceived as amateurs, dilettantes. The military was not favorable to newcomers, particularly ones with no credentials. Fielding a new and unknown substance meant taking on entrenched fiefdoms and the inevitable old boys' club. Dacorta found himself feeling almost protective of Bart and Frank. And there was a potential concern. Just as Frank had discovered in his early testing at the hospital, Dacorta and Alam found that the application of zeolite created heat. They had measured the temperature of the tissue surrounding the pig's wound and found that it got to 50 or 60 degrees Celsius, the equivalent of 140 degrees Fahrenheit. Not exactly scalding, but certainly hot. Also, Dacorta said that QuikClot would likely be messy at times to use on the battlefield. In high winds in the desert of Iraq, the granules of zeolite might fly away across the sands. Once applied, the mineral would have to be washed out of the injury site before the wound was stitched up. Dacorta told Bart and Frank that the army might someday use these things against them. "In fact, be prepared for it," he said.

But when QuikClot was deployed in Iraq, Dacorta soon began hearing from marines and navy personnel that the product was performing spectacularly well in the field. He also heard stories of army soldiers bartering with their navy and marine brethren to acquire QuikClot, as well as British soldiers trading liquor to get it. Even army medics contacted him, asking him to "please send us the QuikClot." Dacorta personally packed up cartons of the stuff and sent them to the Middle East. But Dacorta—ever the skeptic—wanted to hear from a doctor or medic who had actually used the stuff on the battlefield. Reports and anecdotes were one thing, direct experience another. He had staked his entire career on what worked—and what did not—in actual combat.

CHAPTER SIX

Already Dead

IN FEBRUARY 2003, Lieutenant Commander Timothy Coakley of the United States Navy was riding shotgun in a Humvee traveling across the deserts of southern Iraq. The Humvee was being driven by a marine corporal under Coakley's command, and the vehicle was part of a large convoy of cargo trucks and Humvees heading toward Baghdad. Suddenly the radio system crackled to life. The convoy commander said in rushed tones that a marine in a truck half a mile ahead had been shot in the neck.

Within minutes Coakley and his driver found the cargo truck pulled over by the side of the road. Coakley exited his vehicle. Lying on the ground was a tall, blond, blue-eyed marine, a private, looking more like a high schooler than a soldier, gasping for air and writhing in agony. Blood spouted out of his neck. He was in full combat gear—tan boots, head-to-toe camo, body armor, helmet— and the blood was staining his chest and legs in dark, ever-widening crimson circles. A medic knelt over the fallen marine, hyperventilating and saying, "Oh my God! Oh my God!" over and over again.

Coakley knew the type—clearly the medic was a reservist who had never dreamed he would actually see combat. Two of the fallen marine's fellow soldiers stood nearby, mute. Coakley examined the young marine and saw that for the moment, anyway, he was lucky. A sniper's bullet had passed through the marine's neck but had narrowly missed his windpipe and carotid artery. Still, the solider was losing a great deal of blood, and quickly.

"You can get out of here," Coakley instructed the medic. "I am an emergency physician. I've got this." Coakley instructed the medic to call for a military ambulance. Then he got on his knees and went to work.

It was in these moments that things always slowed down for him. Coakley retrieved surgical gloves and compressed gauze from his medical kit. "It's gonna be OK," he told the prone solider. He depressed the gauze into the gaping cavities in the soldier's neck, one in the front and one in the back. The marine remained conscious but wore a stunned expression, looking stoically up toward the sky. He breathed in agonized fits and starts. The gauze slowed the bleeding, but not much; the flow of blood was still voluminous. Coakley knew he needed to find a solution quickly, or the soldier was at risk of bleeding out. They were in the middle of the desert, and it might be some time—ten, twenty, thirty minutes—before an ambulance arrived.

Coakley rifled through his medical kit. Inside he found a small beige pouch labeled "QuikClot." He remembered a predeployment training three months earlier at Camp Lejeune in North Carolina in which a medic had explained that QuikClot was a brand-new product capable of stopping big bleeds. Coakley had been highly skeptical. He'd spent the early part of his career, before he got his medical degree, as a navy-enlisted corpsman, or medic, and as an operating room technician. Even in the controlled environment of

the operating room, Coakley had seen that nothing was particularly good at stopping large quantities of blood. But in the desert,
as he knelt next to the marine, he'd said—perhaps foolishly—that
everything was going to be OK. Coakley had no other options. He
glanced at the product directions, opened the packet, and poured
its contents into the hole in the marine's neck before applying more
gauze. Then Coakley waited, expecting nothing, a sinking feeling
growing in his stomach that the soldier's life hung in the balance.

And nothing happened at first, but then, after ten seconds, it
appeared to Coakley that the blood began to slow. After twenty
seconds, Coakley clearly saw the blood thickening into a kind of
dark-crimson Jell-O. And then, in the next minute, the bleeding
effectively ceased. Coakley packed more gauze into the wounds,
and this time he was able to fully control the excess bleeding. It
was as if a clot had formed in front of his eyes. *Holy shit*, Coakley
thought, *the military finally came up with something that works. I can't
fucking believe it.* "You're going to be all right," Coakley said to the
marine, this time with conviction. He held the gauze in place until
the military ambulance, a modified Humvee with a red cross on
it, arrived twenty minutes later. Coakley helped lift the marine into
the ambulance and watched as the Humvee drove away toward a
nearby surgical company, gradually disappearing across the desert.
He thought the marine would survive, but you could never know
for sure. Whatever this QuikClot was, Coakley mused, it had
promise. But then again, he thought, anything could work once, its
success never to be repeated—particularly in combat.

Coakley had been in Iraq and Kuwait for three months, even
though the war hadn't officially started yet. He was the leader of
one of the marines' twenty-four so-called Shock Trauma platoons
deployed in the run-up to the conflict. Coakley's platoon, part of the
Second Marine Logistic Group of the Second Medical Battalion,

was comprised of twenty-five marines, including a dentist, a nurse, medics, electricians, drivers, and security personnel. The platoon's primary mission was to assist in the implementation of the medical supply chain for the impending war. Coakley had spent the last three months barely sleeping, overseeing the process by which the correct supplies for the imminently arriving medical units— syringes, bandages, drugs, surgical gloves, cots, blankets, and so on—got to the base camp in Kuwait and were dispatched via cargo truck to combat hospitals and field locations in Iraq.

Coakley had first arrived in Kuwait right after Christmas 2002, a few days after his fortieth birthday, leaving his wife and five children behind in Virginia. Mainly he had been stationed at the Kuwait Naval Base and Camp Fox, a logistical base camp for the marines just outside of Kuwait City. Both of these locations served as staging areas as the American military prepared for war. Camp Fox, where he spent most of his time, seemed less like a place than a random stopping point in the desert. It was effectively a large tent city with a massive barbed-wire fence around it. Inside the compound were smaller individual tent cities, each encircled by its own barbed-wire fence. But mostly Camp Fox was made up of hundreds upon hundreds of various types of vehicles as well as CONEX shipping containers, acres and acres of them. Beyond the perimeter of Camp Fox was simply desert, punctuated by flocks of sheep and the occasional donkey or camel. In the daytime the sands took on an almost apocalyptic orange color, while at night there were black clouds on the horizon and what appeared to be the glow of fire. Were those oil fires? No one seemed to know. The temperatures were beastly in their extremes—it could rise to 110 degrees during the day and then become shockingly cold at night. The heat was so intense that Coakley and his platoon members would pour a small puddle of water on top of a metal drum and then make bets about how long it would take for it to evaporate. Sometimes it was just minutes. The whole place carried with it a feeling of infinite desolation. Once the invasion of Iraq started, Coakley spent two months traveling back and forth between Kuwait and Iraq, the nearly daily convoys comprised of dozens of thirty-foot tractor trailers. Medical supplies were a small part of the freight. Most of the trucks carried food, water, and weapons.

A few weeks after treating the blond marine, Coakley was part of another convoy. This was a larger and longer mission, a three-day journey to Baghdad. It was late afternoon, and Coakley was traveling in a line of trucks and Humvees along a meandering avenue that led into a suburb of Baghdad. The four-lane road was lined with palm trees and with shops and houses and schools made from stucco and concrete. Coakley heard but never saw the bomb. Even in the tightly sealed confines of his Humvee, with its bullet-resistant windshield, the sound was frightening. In the ensuing chaos, it was unclear exactly where the bomb had detonated, and his driver kept moving forward. The chatter immediately commenced on the radio: "Holy fucking shit: a bomb went off!" Coakley was instructed to look for casualties. A block later, after crossing a bridge, Coakley spotted a man lying on the sidewalk, an Iraqi civilian who was bleeding badly and crying out. Coakley got out of his vehicle and saw that a large portion of the man's back had been ripped open. The man was dazed but conscious. Coakley could see that there was no shrapnel embedded in the wounds, but he knew that there didn't have to be shrapnel for there to be damage. By this time Coakley had been in war zones long enough to know that the initial blast of an improvised explosive device, or IED, did not always inflict the most carnage. The greater part of the damage of an IED was often meted out by the second or third or even fourth blast wave, all of which were generated by the vacuum and overpressure of compressed air created by the first. The subsequent waves produced hurricane-like forces capable of eviscerating and even amputating body parts. Kneeling by the man, Coakley knew that the flesh of his back had been ripped off by those secondary blast waves.

The man's bleeding was copious, the blood running in rivulets down the sidewalk. Coakley ripped open two packets of QuikClot and poured their contents into the wound. The blood once again congealed until the massive wound could be controlled simply with gauze. Coakley tried to assure the man that everything was going to be OK, even though neither spoke the other's language. It took a full two hours for an Iraqi ambulance to arrive. Coakley sat with the man the whole time.

While he waited, Coakley wondered what it was about QuikClot that made it such an effective blood clotting agent. It was a little like science fiction. He resolved that whenever the war was over, if he survived, he would study QuikClot in the labs at the Naval Hospital Portsmouth back home.

No one had ever expected Timothy Coakley to amount to much, let alone become a doctor and a lieutenant commander in the navy—the equivalent of a major in the army. He barely graduated from high school. A month before graduation, he told one of the nuns at his Catholic high school of his plans to join the navy and become a medic. She responded, "That's good, but just remember, when you get out of the service, the world will still need ditchdiggers."

A self-described "short, fat kid," Coakley grew up in a blue-collar town near Chicago where his father worked at the Caterpillar tractor factory. He was close to his mother and his three siblings, but he was bullied by his father and demeaned by his grandfather, and he struggled academically. In high school he was known equally for his mediocre grades—mainly Cs—and the gameness of his spirit. He got into fistfights in the schoolyard and despite his size—five foot seven—played offensive guard and tackle on the football team.

But the navy turned out to be a good fit for Coakley. Growing up, he had almost certainly suffered from undiagnosed attention deficit hyperactivity disorder, and the structure and discipline of the service were ideal for him. Showing a long-latent aptitude, he began to excel at anatomy, biology, and chemistry in his coursework. He received specialized training in undersea and barometric medicine in Connecticut. He went on to become an operating room technician at the Naval Hospital Corps School in Illinois. He also volunteered for the occasional special mission. In the mid-1980s the Reagan administration periodically conducted military exercises in Honduras as part of a show of force for the leftist government of Nicaragua. Coakley volunteered to be a corpsman on a surgical team aboard the USS *Nassau*, an amphibious assault ship carrying three thousand personnel, on a three-week mission in the Caribbean Sea. One night, he went out into the bay with a group of navy SEALs in rigid inflatable boats. Suddenly an unfamiliar boat approached them through the dark. The SEALs warned off the nearing boat with instructions from a megaphone and shots fired in the air, but the mysterious craft kept coming toward them. At the last moment, the boat peeled away into the night. It was a tense moment, but afterward Coakley realized that he had found the episode strangely exhilarating.

In his early twenties Coakley enrolled in community college while still working full-time at the hospital. At the start of the semester he proclaimed to his old high school classmates that someday he was going to become a doctor. No one believed him. In fact, the administrators at the college were so suspicious of Coakley—based on his high school transcript—that they placed him on academic probation even before his first class. But he completed the first and second year with straight A's and transferred to Northern Illinois University, where he got his bachelor's degree in three years, taking night and summer school classes. School, especially biology and chemistry, now came easily to him. It was as if a switch had been flipped on. He could easily visualize formulas and molecules and neurons. The quickness and jumpiness of his mind, which for so long had been hindrances, were now assets. In his junior year of college, he married and started a family. He was accepted to Chicago Medical School, graduating in 1995 and inducted into the Alpha Omega Alpha academic fraternity, reserved for the top 15 percent of medical students nationally. When it came to choosing a specialty, there was no question that he was going to go into emergency medicine. It had the most action and the quickest pace, and it suited his restless nature. He did his internship at a marines base camp in California, did advanced training as an undersea medical officer, and was subsequently assigned to the navy's special operations forces in both deep-sea diving and explosive ordnance disposal—the detecting and disarming of bombs in extreme environments. He went on to become chief resident at the Naval Hospital Portsmouth, Virginia, the oldest and largest of the navy hospitals. His patients, mainly navy personnel and their families, never ceased to comment that Dr. Coakley was different from any other doctor they knew: he had no pretense, no ego, and engaged in no bullshit. He was a regular guy who happened to have a medical degree.

Coakley was in the emergency room at the naval hospital on Thanksgiving 2002 when he got the call that he was going to be deployed in a month's time first to Kuwait and then later to Iraq to lead the Shock Trauma platoon. But first he was told to report to Camp Lejeune, the Marine Corps training facility in North Carolina. Coakley was not particularly upset about going off to war—after 9/11 it appeared that a conflict in the Middle East was inevitable—but he left the States feeling unsettled. He and his wife had been struggling for some time, and his five kids were now entering a critical period of their young lives.

During those first few months at Camp Fox, Coakley—like Joe Dacorta before him, when Dacorta was overseeing medical logistics during the Gulf War—was stunned by the shabby state of the equipment and supplies that the military provided its marines. The uniform he was given had holes in it, and his boots were used. But that was nothing compared to the shortcomings of the medical supplies. The tubes for medical intubation were cracked. The bandages were yellowed and frayed, as if they were from the Vietnam, or even the World War II, era. And there simply weren't enough of them. At one point in Iraq, Coakley's colleagues were reduced to using underwear and socks to bandage a soldier. Nor were there sufficient weapons or body armor for medical personnel. Even cell phones and radios were lacking or faulty. Coakley soon realized that the abject state of the supplies was a particular problem of the marines—not so much the army, which mainly had the latest in everything. The marines seemed to get only the hand-me-downs. Coakley began to think of the marines as the bastard child of the service branches. While visiting an army base camp, he observed amenities such as a food court with a Burger King, a Pizza Hut, and a Starbucks, a fitness center, ATMs, and even recreation areas with a game room, free snacks, and movie nights.

At Camp Fox, Coakley repeatedly lobbied the logistic officers, saying he needed more and better equipment. He had been given a "table of allowances" of equipment, which promised him a specific amount of what his platoon needed to function, everything from personnel to body armor to rifles to vehicles to generators. Most of the time he did not receive what he had been promised. His initial allotment of equipment was about 20 percent of what he had been expecting. "We are going to war!" he screamed at the logistics people. "My group is going to be among the first ones in." The logistics officers began to ignore him. Many of them were reservists and thought the Iraqi conflict was going to be Desert Storm all over again. It would be over in a month. They would put in a handful of weeks, get their credit, go home. It would be like hanging out at the beach, only in the desert. "Don't worry," they would tell Coakley. Using military jargon to indicate they were planning on just coasting by, far from the action, they said, "Hey, man, we are just swinging the wings, in the rear with the gear."

Coakley decided to take matters into his own hands. He didn't care if he had to lie, cheat, or steal to get his comrades their due. Since he had been among the first of the marine medical personnel to arrive in the Middle East, and had the most—in the language of the marines—"ground intel" about how things worked, or rather didn't work, he became known around the base as "1-800-Coakley" or simply "411," the man who could get you anything. The way he thought about it was that he had twenty-five marines and medical personnel under him, and he was responsible for their lives. Since they were going to be among the first into Iraq, no one knew what lay head of them.

Coakley was even able to procure alcohol. He told the medical supply officers that he needed booze because it was a known antidote to the toxins of antifreeze. It was not uncommon for desperate marines to attempt suicide by drinking antifreeze. Even relatively small amounts can be fatal, but alcohol can reverse the effects of the toxins on the kidneys. Eventually the footlocker in his tent contained choice bottles of Jack Daniel's, Bacardi, and Johnnie Walker Red. Coakley observed that some Iraqis had a special fascination with Johnnie Walker in particular, and he developed a habit of carrying a small bottle of it in his backpack. One night Coakley was in a Humvee near Baghdad when he and his driver came to a fork in the road. The maps and the intelligence they had been given were unclear. Should they go left or should they go right? The wrong decision could kill them. There were many Iraqi locals loyal to Saddam Hussein's Republican Guard who would be very interested in setting a US Navy officer and his convoy crew down the wrong road into a potential ambush. As they sat at the side of the road figuring out the best option, Coakley spotted an Iraqi man. Coakley had a feeling about the guy. He got out of the Humvee alongside his interpreter and asked him for directions. As he did so, he pulled out the Johnnie Walker bottle and handed it to the man. "That way," the man said. Coakley and his fellow marines completed the trip without incident. A bottle of whiskey may have saved his life.

Four months into his tour, Coakley volunteered to provide medical support on a two-day mission. Once again he rode as a passenger in a convoy of Humvees and tractor trailers. It was three in the morning, and he had been up for thirty-six hours. In an instant Coakley's vehicle was rocked by an explosion. The two tractor trailers ahead of him stopped and came under fire. Pieces of them flew into the air. Coakley was blown out of the Humvee and landed in the middle of the road, stunned and woozy, the blast ringing in his ears. Shots were being fired all around him. In the midst of the chaos, he saw a lizard dash across the road. *I wish I was that lizard*, he thought. As he came to, he took a quick inventory of his body: nothing appeared to be broken, but he was certain he had a concussion. A marine dragged him to cover behind one of the trucks. "Why are you saving me? Aren't others hurt more badly?" Coakley shouted at him. "Because you're the doc. We need you!" the soldier shouted back.

Coakley would end up spending another five months in Iraq, and although he was never directly hit, he was in close proximity to exploding IEDs on a number of occasions. The sonic forces of the secondary blast waves were terrifying and led to headaches, numbness, and blurred vision. Still, Coakley was unwilling to say no to special missions. Sometimes he was pulled into high-security tasks by the State Department and saw unimaginable horrors: the bodies of dead children, decapitated heads on the ground, corpses stacked like cordwood. The more time he spent in Iraq, the more things became a timeless jumble of sleeplessness, exhaustion, and tedium, of sweat and filth and fear combined with almost im-measurable relief at having survived another encounter with the terrifying whiz of bullets and the bursting of shells. And there was just the constant insane tableau of the war, day after day: soldiers defecating in the desert, children selling bottles of water along the roadside, dogs with three legs, concertina wire around everything, craters in the earth left by bombs, burned-out tanks. He was on a tour of a doomed world, as if in some deranged movie.

He also realized that what kept everybody going was the sacred bond that existed among all the members of his platoon. He would tell his charges, "This is the way you have to look at it—you are already dead. That way if you survive, it is just a blessing, icing on the cake. Unexpected. Assume you are already dead, and you have nothing to lose." It was this shared ethos that kept them together. But at the same time, no one was quite sure what they were doing there, other than adhering to vague notions of freedom. They liked to believe that they were liberating a country from a dictator, but they had little evidence to show for it. Actually, every day it was the opposite: seeing dead people and wounds and bombs in such random configurations made it difficult to believe there was any center or coherence to this mission at all. Everything was shadows, subterfuge. Nothing could be trusted. Underneath it all, Coakley seethed with anger that the military hadn't backed the common soldiers up with what they needed. And he had this increasingly foreboding sense that things were not going to be good at home when he returned. Communication with his wife had slowed to rare, progressively more awkward phone calls and email exchanges.

In late July he was abruptly called back to the United States with only three days' notice. That was the military—you did what you were told. He left so hastily that he was still in combat gear, with blood on his boots, and carrying only a rucksack when he boarded the airplane. Everyone else on the flight was a combatant returning from the war. They flew from Kuwait to Germany, where they refueled, to Washington, D.C., and on to the Marine Corps Air Station in Cherry Point, North Carolina. On the plane Coakley drank Scotch. He couldn't sleep. Guilt weighed heavily on him. He had survived the war after all, but he was leaving his marines behind to meet whatever fate lay ahead of them. He felt horrible about leaving. When he called his family upon arrival, his wife said she couldn't meet him at Cherry Point as all the other soldiers' families were doing. "The kids are tired," she said. He knew in that moment that his marriage was over. From Cherry Point he took a bus to Camp Lejeune, a sixty-mile trip toward the coast. He was instructed to go to the central issue facility to turn his gear in. He barely noticed the marine private who took his equipment. But he heard the young man's voice, which was strained and scratchy. And then he noticed the marine's neck and saw the Z-shaped scar on it. The private looked down at Coakley. He was tall, blue eyed, and blond. The private's eyes grew large with recognition, and he grabbed Coakley by his shoulders. Tears welled up in the private's eyes. "You're the one," the marine said. "You're the one who said I would make it when I was shot in the neck. It was you. Thank you. Thank you." Coakley was so numb, so overcome with emotion, that all he could say was, "Wow. My God, you're welcome."

After he turned in his gear, Coakley went to a liquor store with two men in his platoon who had flown home with him. The three bought a bottle of rum and sat on a curb until they passed out. He had earlier called for a driver from the Naval Hospital Portsmouth, who then picked him up and drove him to Virginia. On the long ride home, Coakley kept thinking about the encounter with the blond marine who had thanked him for saving his life. Coakley had no idea what the last eight months had all meant, but it was clear that he had accomplished one tangible thing during his time in the fog of war—something that no one could ever take away from him. He had helped save a desperate young man who had been in the shadows of death. All Coakley kept thinking was, *I may have saved that marine's life, but he saved mine tonight.*

The following Monday, he was supposed to report to the Emergency Department at the hospital at Portsmouth to see patients. He couldn't face the idea of returning to work and asked the hospital for a two-week leave. He was told no leaves were being issued for returning physicians.

He reported to work as scheduled and saw his supervisor, the director of the Emergency Department, for the first time in eight months. Coakley had lost thirty-five pounds and did not look well.

"What the hell happened to you?" she asked.

"I've seen stuff you wouldn't believe. What can I say? It was a shit show," Coakley replied. "If you insist that I work in the

ER, I promise you that I will be the most dangerous physician on the floor."

She granted him the leave immediately.

Tensions were high at home, so Coakley moved into a five-hundred-square-foot apartment near Norfolk above a garage. Behind the garage was a large yard bounded by a river. He lived there for the next six months, trying to recover from whatever had happened to him in Iraq.

Not long after he returned, Coakley was contacted by Joe Dacorta. Dacorta had sent a group email to navy doctors and medics inquiring if they had used QuikClot in the field and, if so, what their experience had been. Coakley already knew Dacorta from the fairly close circles of marine medicine. Three years earlier they had done a presentation together at a military medicine conference in Tampa Bay. Coakley called Dacorta.

"Did you use QuikClot in the field?" Dacorta asked.

"Did I ever!" Coakley said. "That stuff is fantastic!"

"Would you be willing to speak about your experiences with it?" He told Coakley that in two weeks there was going to be a special operations medical conference, focusing on trauma medicine, in Florida, and all the bigwigs would be there. There would be sessions on QuikClot, HemCon, and other new products that had recently been introduced into the theater of war.

"Of course," Coakley said. "I would love to. Finally the military discovered something that worked."

A few weeks later, Coakley found himself behind a lectern in a large conference room in the Tradewinds Hotel in St. Petersburg. He wore a full-dress uniform: a white cap with a gold-and-navy visor, navy blue hard shoulder boards with three gold stripes each, a gold star with a single acorn indicating his service in the Medical Corps, and combat medals on his chest. He had flown in the night before from Virginia and met up with Dacorta. The Tradewinds was a massive beachfront hotel on eighteen acres overlooking the Gulf of Mexico. There he briefly met Bart Gullong. It was 95 degrees outside and sweltering. Bart was sweating by the pool. Coakley thought he looked a bit like a pirate. "Thank you for what you are doing. I really appreciate it," Bart said. Bart said that unfortunately he couldn't attend the session because he had to man the QuikClot product booth on the exhibit floor. Dacorta escorted Coakley to a large plenary session room, where a crowd of about fifty was filing in.

Coakley expected that his remarks would be received well, that the session would amount to a kind of victory lap, as he would be one of the first emissaries from the battlefield to deliver the news of the military's major medical breakthrough. But he sensed an odd atmosphere from the beginning. A good portion of the crowd refused to even sit down. They stood warily along the back wall even though there were plenty of seats. Coakley later learned that these were army doctors, medics, representatives of HemCon, and employees of North American Rescue, the company that distributed HemCon. They seemed angry, ready for a fight, almost as if they were part of a gang.

Coakley began his story about using QuikClot on the marine shot in the neck. "I couldn't believe how well it stopped the bleeding in its tracks," he said. "This product was amazing. Before I became a doctor, I worked as an operating room tech, and nothing was ever any good at clotting large amounts of blood. I never thought the field of medicine would find something that worked so well, let alone the navy and marines discovering it—"

"How do you know it worked?" interjected one of the men in the back.

"Umm…because I saw it with my own eyes," Coakley said. "And because the marine survived."

Coakley went on to the second story, about the Iraqi civilian whose back was ripped open by the bomb.

"That was remarkable too," he said. "To see the zeolite absorb so much blood showed me that the first time wasn't a fluke. I knew we really had something here—"

"What are you implying?" another man in the back said. "That the army drop HemCon and take on a whole new product which requires extensive training?"

"That is *exactly* what I am implying. Besides, it doesn't require extensive training," Coakley responded.

"But what about the directions for use?" someone asked.

"I read the directions only seconds before I used it. Just don't eat it, as it says on the package. That's just about the only training that is required!"

Many in the crowd laughed. None of the men standing in the back did.

"But don't you know that QuikClot burns people?" an army doctor shouted at him.

Coakley said he had seen the blood get hot when he added QuikClot, but it was nothing that he considered serious, especially given the product's benefits. "I will tell you right now," Coakley said. "Soldiers in combat will sign up for a little burn any day of the week. When your life is on the line, this is the stuff you want."

After the speech, Coakley was surrounded at the lectern by the army doctors and HemCon reps.

"What do you know?" one man asked.

"You're not a researcher!" another yelled.

"You're not from the Institute of Surgical Research! You're not from the army!" a third person said.

Coakley felt himself becoming incensed. "You're damn right I'm not from the army. I am a navy doctor and former medic and I just came back from eight months in combat and I used this stuff personally," Coakley said. "By the way, when was the last time you were in combat?"

Finally Dacorta intervened, escorting Coakley to the relative safety of the hotel lobby. There were still a large group of people out there. A number of them, navy medics and doctors mainly, congratulated and thanked Coakley. But the army and HemCon reps continued to crowd him uncomfortably.

On the periphery of what was beginning to feel almost like a skirmish, a tall, distinguished-looking man with slightly graying hair stood quietly, saying nothing. Something about him seemed important, and in the confusion of the moment, Coakley reached out to shake his hand. The man spurned the gesture and walked away. An older, very short and slight man in a suit lingered quietly in a corner, observing the whole scene. After everyone left, he approached Coakley and gave him his business card. "I like what you're doing, Dr. Coakley," the man said. "But do you know who you are dealing with? You're playing with the big boys now. If you ever have any trouble, I want you to give me a call."

Coakley took the card and looked at it. The man was a senior official from the Office of Health Affairs at the Department of Defense. That is, the Pentagon. Coakley put the card in his wallet.

That night, Coakley and Dacorta met on the beach. A band was playing reggae music. "You set me up, man," Coakley said to Dacorta, laughingly. "That was a fucking ambush you put me into."

"What can I say?" Dacorta said, smiling. "I heard you were a scrappy Irishman. I figured you'd be able to handle it."

"That was like I was Jimmy Stewart in *Mr. Smith Goes to Washington*," Coakley said. "If I wasn't a little drunk right now, I'd say fuck you."

"It couldn't be worse than enemy fire," Dacorta said.

"I'm not so sure about that," Coakley laughed. "By the way, who the fuck was that guy who wouldn't even shake my hand?"

"That's Dr. John Holcomb, a colonel and head of trauma medicine for the army," Dacorta said.

The more Coakley reflected on it, the more furious he became about the Tradewinds conference. In the moment he had been more stunned than anything else, but as he tried to reestablish a routine back home in Virginia, he became more incensed. *How dare Holcomb and his minions treat me that way?* All his life he had been doubted and shown up by people like Holcomb. The army doctors had refuted his actual experience as if it had never happened.

Coakley returned to work as an emergency physician at the Naval Hospital Portsmouth, but on days off he would drive to Quantico to meet with Dacorta, Given, and Eagles. When the four of them went out to dinner one night in Quantico, Eagles took Coakley aside. He said, "Son, I know you just came back and I can smell the combat on you. I've been there. I will pray for you. And if you ever need any help, call me anytime." Coakley never did call Eagles, but he was glad of the offer. At these meetings Coakley also told Dacorta and Given that he wanted to learn more about QuikClot. As a medical student he had taken a particular interest in the blood clotting cascade, and he wondered whether there might be something behind QuikClot's remarkable efficacy beyond its absorption of water. Coakley thought that zeolite might additionally work by directly affecting the proteins in the clotting cascade. He also thought the electrical charges in zeolite might be a factor. He threw around these ideas with Dacorta, who was impressed by Coakley's acumen. As Dacorta put it later, "Tim was not a conventional scientist, but he was great at asking questions of the universe." Over the course of a few months, Coakley raised the notion of conducting more advanced research on QuikClot under Dacorta's and Given's auspices, and he undertook the arduous process of submitting research proposals to do so to the Office of Naval Research, the National Institutes of Health, and the Navy Surgeon General, all of which were eventually approved. He set up a lab in the Naval Hospital Portsmouth and began testing QuikClot on pigs.

About six months after returning from the war, Coakley began experiencing increased migraines and problems moving his fingers to perform suturing. He often felt numb and was sometimes disoriented and confused. He barely slept at night. Gory scenes of combat ran constantly through his head. When he did sleep, he often woke up in a startled state. He found himself crying at a moment's notice, sometimes about nothing at all. Coakley, the combat doctor, knew full well that his symptoms were likely linked to traumatic brain injury from his continued exposure to explosive devices in Iraq. But he also thought he could just muscle through. The turning point came one day in the emergency room when Coakley attempted to suture a complex laceration on the face of a ten-year-old girl who had been bitten by a dog. It was a traumatic, if not ultimately a serious, wound. Normally it would have taken Coakley an hour to complete the stitches, but his hands were shaking so much that it took him three hours. After a month of extensive testing, evidence of neurological damage was detected in his brain, and he entered the neurotherapy rehabilitation program at the University of Virginia hospital, where he did dexterity and memory exercises, often on the computer, and worked with a physical rehabilitation therapist. He also joined a group therapy session for veterans of combat. All of these things helped, but especially the group therapy. Coakley found that only those who had also "been there" could understand what he was going through.

His other therapy was working on QuikClot in the hospital lab at night. He had been stunned by the effectiveness of zeolite and wanted to better understand how the rock worked so well at clotting blood. He also wanted to experiment with different proportions of zeolite and blood in order to find the optimal ratio for clotting while keeping heat down. He had excelled in medical school, but he believed his new insights were on another level. Now he constantly started to see scientific images in his mind, like the molecular structure of zeolite, just as Frank Hursey had twenty years earlier. They were like visions, or hallucinations, exhilarating but also a little scary and extreme. But after all the suffering, it was exciting—thrilling, even—to finally be making something out of his experience. Years later, he speculated that he may have during this period developed savant syndrome, a phenomenon whereby a person who has recovered from traumatic brain injury enters an unexpected period of creativity. It was as if his brain had been shocked into a primitive state from all the exposure to bombs and had then reemerged in a more advanced state. The research kept him going. With his family life in wreckage and his psyche mired in trauma, unlocking the secrets that lay within zeolite was about the only good thing in his life.

The war in Iraq was now in full force, and two or three times a year, various branches of the military held conferences around the country to discuss innovations in battlefield medicine. Dacorta, Coakley, and Bart always attended these events—even if Bart rarely got to the actual sessions, as he was almost always working the booth in the exhibit hall, usually in the basement. Coakley, both motivated and emboldened by the hostile reception to his first presentation at the Tradewinds, volunteered to make presentations about his experiences with QuikClot at these conferences and also began conducting trainings on how best to use the product at military bases around the country. He was fervent about spreading the word about QuikClot and getting it into the hands of as many soldiers as possible, including those in the army. The lives of "the kids in the ditch"—as Tom Eagles always said—were at stake, and Coakley felt personally responsible for helping to save them.

His research into QuikClot was progressing nicely, and a public affairs officer in the navy's Bureau of Medicine and Surgery suggested that he write a letter to the Republican senator from Virginia, John Warner, to pursue additional funding. Coakley was his constituent, and Warner was chair of the Senate Armed Services Committee and had been under secretary of the navy under Nixon. The public affairs officer coached Coakley in writing the letter and how to describe his work. It was now September 2004, a couple of months before the Bush/Kerry election, which was shaping up to be a referendum on the Iraq War. In the last couple of months, Coakley had been interviewed on television networks and media outlets about his combat experience and use of QuikClot. Of course Bart and Frank were only too happy to have an actual combat veteran speak about their product.

Coakley was in the hospital in October 2004 when he received a call from a navy captain in the office of his commanding officer who informed him that a formal preliminary court-martial investigation was being initiated against him. The captain said that soliciting military funding directly from a member of Congress was a violation of military law in the navy, something of which Coakley had been unaware. The captain went on to say that there was going to be a preliminary hearing in a few days with Coakley's commanding officer, Rear Admiral Thomas Burkhard, commander of the Naval Hospital Portsmouth, to review the allegations. Coakley was stunned because he believed he had gone through all the proper channels. As he tried to put things together, he became convinced he had been set up by the public affairs officer and that surely she wouldn't have been acting alone; she would have been instructed and directed by someone from the upper echelons of navy medicine. He couldn't know for sure, but he began to think that someone was trying to shut down the rogue doctor who spoke his mind publicly, and suspected that it had all begun with his remarks at the Tradewinds.

In this conversation the captain also asked Coakley if he had received the proper permissions to do his research. Coakley said he had gotten approvals from all the proper authorities ahead of time. He went to his computer at the hospital to print them out and was stunned to find that his emails had been deleted off his server. Now he was starting to get even more paranoid—or maybe not paranoid; he believed he was being targeted. Coakley immediately called the IT Department at the hospital, with which he was friendly. Coakley had always treated the staff there like his peers, unlike many of the doctors, and offered them medical advice when they'd asked. They restored the emails, and Coakley printed out all the documents immediately, proving that he'd followed procedures, and put everything in a three-inch-thick binder. This turned out to be a wise decision, because the next day his emails mysteriously disappeared again. Someone very high up was after him, Coakley now felt certain.

Right after the conversation with the captain, Coakley called the official from the Pentagon who had given his card to Coakley after the Tradewinds presentation. They met at a deli in Arlington, Virginia. "I think I'm in trouble," Coakley said. "I think you were right. The big boys came after me."

The official didn't say much, but he promised he would make some calls. "Things will work out," the Pentagon man said. "Let me see what I can do."

The hearing—although it was never officially called that, nor was Coakley ever informed of a specific charge or given anything in writing—was in Admiral Burkhard's office a few days later. At the meeting was Burkhard, the navy captain who had informed him of the allegations, the public affairs officer Coakley believed had set him up, and a judicial advocate, who would represent Coakley. Coakley brought the emails with him. When he was accused of not following research procedures, Coakley showed everyone present the emails, which demonstrated he had. They reviewed the papers and dropped the matter.

Then Burkhard asked about the solicitation of funds.

Coakley said, "I had no idea that was out of bounds, sir. I was unaware of that. This was all new territory for me."

The captain then asked Coakley to leave the room while the others had a conference call with a senior official in navy medicine. This also came as a shock to Coakley.

Coakley waited in the hall, sweating profusely.

He could hear raised voices coming from the office. He couldn't make out much, but he heard a voice screaming, "I want him fucking out of the navy!" Some more discussion ensued; Coakley couldn't make out the words.

A few minutes later, Coakley was asked back into the office.

Burkhard said, "You are the luckiest sailor in the navy, Commander Coakley. We are not going further with this. And by the way, I like what you are doing."

Coakley left the room, vindicated but also confused. He found out later from the judicial advocate what had happened during the call. The man at the top had wanted Coakley gone, but the public affairs officer had mentioned that Coakley had been in the national media lately, talking about his experiences in Iraq. The Bush/Kerry election was in a few weeks, and if they moved forward with court-martial procedures, the officials feared Coakley could become even more of a loose cannon, going to the media about things he'd seen in Iraq or how he'd been treated. That was when the navy backed off.

Coakley was relieved, to be sure, but he also felt he couldn't trust anyone. No matter his service on the battlefield, he was the rogue doctor, the outsider who'd gone to community college, always the black sheep. Coakley had been in combat and would be again in the future; all told, he would serve a year and a half in combat, not just in Iraq but also in later missions around the world. The elite doctors still thought of him as the short, fat kid from Chicago.

Coakley believed it all to be a conspiracy—really, part of the image that had followed him his whole life: that he was an underdog, the guy who talked too fast, shot from the hip, didn't follow protocol, and could be dismissed at any time. He didn't mind not being part of the club; he was proud of his work and his service. But what he couldn't get over when he looked back on this time—and would never get over—was that he felt the army in particular had called into question his actual, lived experience treating wounded patients under enemy fire on foreign soil. It filled him with limitless and withering anger.

And that, to Coakley, was worse than combat itself.

CHAPTER SEVEN

"You burn people!"

BY THE TIME Bart Gullong met Tim Coakley at the Tradewinds Hotel in August 2003 he was feeling better about himself than he had for years. The emotional crater he had found himself in before he met Frank—those years in the Hamptons, all that wasted time, those hangovers and lost relationships—seemed firmly and neatly in the past. Financially he had exceeded even his own expectations. Bart had worked with Frank for four years by this point and was now earning a remarkable $800,000 a year. Frank was making even more than that.

In fact Bart had achieved just what he had set out to do in returning to his home state of Connecticut, the Land of Steady Habits. He was providing amply for his family, he had found work that was deeply meaningful to him, and his sense of well-being had returned. His now eight-year-old daughter, Sarah, was thriving, and his relationship with his wife, Linda, was more stable than it had been for some time. They lived in an expansive house in a high-end development of thirty colonial houses in Niantic, a small shore town in eastern Connecticut. Bart took to calling the neighborhood "the Pfizer ghetto" because most of the neighbors were executives and scientists at the pharmaceutical giant, which had a large research and development site nearby. The drive from the Pfizer ghetto to his office in Newington took almost an hour, but to Bart it was worth it. He would gladly commute that distance to have a house near the ocean. In the morning he used the time in the car to plan out the day; on the ride home he decompressed, listening to pop music on the FM radio station out of Hartford.

Bart could measure his recent success by the ever-increasing dimensions of the boat he bought every year. He had graduated from a simple outboard motorboat to a forty-five-foot used yacht. Many weekends, he and Linda and Sarah would sail on Long Island Sound. It was out on the open water where Bart felt most at peace and closest to his family; only there could he escape the constant sales calls, the daily pressure of running a small company, and the punishing amount of air travel that still dominated his weekdays.

In Niantic, Bart and Linda quickly became part of the community, hosting picnics with the neighbors and shopping and eating out on Niantic's scenic Main Street. One December, Bart led a community effort to build a massive *A Christmas Carol*–inspired float for a charity parade to benefit an organization that adopted families in need for the holidays, providing food and presents. To construct the float, Bart managed to borrow Connecticut College rowing trailers, costumes and props from a local theater company, and Styrofoam bricks from a chemical company, and he and his neighbors built an elaborate scene of Bob Cratchit's house on Christmas morning. On the night of the event, as the parade slowly made its way down Main Street, a group of neighbors sat around a big hearth on top of the float, with an actual cooked turkey steaming in the cold air. A kid playing Tiny Tim shouted out to the crowd, "God bless us, every one!" Bart had also talked a maritime supply company into donating metal rigging. Perched at the end of the rigging, flying out over the crowd, was a teenage girl dressed as an angel. Along the side of the float hung a fifty-foot vinyl banner that read "Scrooge adopted a family for Christmas. You can too." The local newspaper ran pictures of the spectacular creation.

Professionally, Frank and Bart were now managing both growing companies, On-Site Gas and Z-Medica. By 2003, On-Site was generating $12 million of revenue a year. The principal driver of this growth was the POGS, the Portable Oxygen Generating System, created for Joe Dacorta's mobile surgical center. It had saved lives on the battlefield, and now first responder and disaster preparedness teams from all over the country were contacting Bart and Frank and ordering the machines, which cost $30,000 each. Even the army had come around and was now a major customer. The army's Medical Research and Materiel Command in Fort Detrick, Maryland, ordered dozens of the POGSs to serve as components of its own version of a mobile battlefield surgical center. Bart traveled to Maryland, where he worked with army engineers, logistical staff, and purchasing personnel. Unlike Bart's experiences with the Institute of Surgical Research, this collaboration proceeded easily and respectfully. It gave Bart hope that one day he might be able to do the same with the army around the adoption of QuikClot.

Around this time Bart and Frank developed, really for the first time, a truly mutual creative partnership. Of course Frank was still the master engineer and Bart the swashbuckling salesman, but now their roles began to blend. Bart, after all, had once been an inventor himself. Starting around 2002, out of the success of the POGS project, Bart and Frank began working out new applications for the 95 percent pure oxygen and nitrogen that Frank and Sanh's machines generated. Oxygen is central to the blowing and creation of glass, and Frank and Bart approached several companies—variously involved in the production of light bulbs, glass tubes for neon lights, and lab instruments—that bought their machines. Learning that the infusion of oxygen into the waters of commercial fish farms boosted the health of fish, they began selling oxygen machines to aquaculture operations. It was well known that nitrogen helps kill bacteria, allowing perishable food items to last much longer. Bart and Frank contracted with purveyors of fruit, coffee, wine, potato chips, and sweets who used nitrogen machines to preserve their products. Similarly, after conducting hundreds of hours of testing on his own, Frank found that when nitrogen is introduced into a liquid, the oxygen level in the liquid is significantly lowered, curbing bacterial and organic growth. After writing a patent for this finding, Bart and Frank contacted companies in various industries—including chemical and pharmaceutical plants, photo labs, and heating, ventilating, and air-conditioning companies—that bought their machines in order to introduce nitrogen into their chemical baths and storage tanks, preventing the growth of algae and bacteria and extending the operating life of the equipment. Perhaps the most daring application they developed was one originated by Bart. His idea was to create a foam saturated with nitrogen that could be used to put out underground fires in coal mines. Frank took Bart's concept and developed a method of introducing a continuous flow of the nitrogen foam into a mine, either through a borehole or by placing the machines in the mine itself. Over time the nitrogen would replace the oxygen and the fire would simply die out. Bart was dismayed to learn that a company in Japan had developed a similar approach, and he told Frank, "I have to go to Japan and talk to them, to see if they will give us a carve-out on their intellectual property."

"Really?" Frank responded. "That sounds expensive." But Bart did take the nineteen-hour flight to Tokyo and talked the Japanese company into giving On-Site the American rights to the technology. The machines On-Site developed helped extinguish the large emergency fires at the Pikeville Mine in Kentucky in 2004 and the Buchanan Mine in Virginia in 2005.

While Bart could often be loud and brash and Frank was typically circumspect and soft-spoken, they shared the same irreverent, even impish, sense of humor. Frank became very excited when he discovered Gary Larson's *Far Side* cartoons and began sharing them with Bart. "Frank, they've only been around for twenty-five years," Bart said. "You're only just learning of them *now?*" They also had essentially the same left-of-center politics. They supported, and with their newfound wealth donated to, the same political candidates. Very occasionally Bart and Frank would travel together, usually to conferences on manufacturing and product development, and Bart would witness another side of Frank emerge. At a laboratory equipment conference in New Orleans, Bart was surprised to discover how much Frank loved the nightlife there. It was he, not Bart, who wanted to stay up late, listen to jazz, and drink too much on Bourbon Street. When they shared a rental car, Bart was shocked by how fast Frank drove, speeding so much that he would miss his exit.

But more than anything, Bart was protective of Frank. He saw in Frank someone who was entirely lacking in artifice. After virtually every business meeting they had with a prospective client, partner, or even competitor, Frank would say, "Well, they seem like nice guys." Frank always thought everyone's motives were honorable, at least until proven otherwise. Bart operated on the opposite assumption. And Frank could sustain his attention during a business meeting for only a limited time. A predictable fifteen minutes or so after a session started, he would essentially stop speaking, disengage, and quite clearly be thinking about other things. Often he would get up from the table, wander off to the coffee maker or some other contraption, and fiddle with it to see how it worked. Accustomed to this, Bart would simply ignore Frank's departure and carry on, even if the other meeting attendees were confused by Frank's behavior. But when things were wrapping up, Frank always returned to the fold, saying, "Well, this is just great. I think you guys got this covered."

Given these inclinations, Frank let Bart run Z-Medica pretty much on his own. However much promise QuikClot had, Frank was largely disengaged from the product once he had invented it. Frank's true passion was being on the factory floor at On-Site, where he adjusted the machines with Sanh and found new applications for oxygen and nitrogen. Z-Medica, for all its notoriety and its promising contracts with the navy and marines, still had relatively modest revenues compared to the parent company. But in 2004, Frank and Bart agreed that Bart would step away from being CEO of Z-Medica so he could get away from the day-to-day operations and concentrate on sales and strategy, which were what he most liked and was most skilled at. Bart was relieved to get away from the pressure of these day-to-day obligations. Frank hired a new CEO, Steven Blascom, who had all the right credentials as a proper engineer. Steven believed that Z-Medica needed to have its own space and moved the company out of Newington and into a newly constructed office and industrial park twenty miles away in Wallingford, a suburban town just north of New Haven. The new building was modern, even sleek. There were roomy, high-ceilinged offices in front for Bart and a recently hired secretary, and in back was a factory floor where, over time, a staff of twenty worked in shifts to prepare the product. Wearing surgical masks and hairnets, white coats and rubber gloves, the workers sterilized the zeolite, which came in barrels from Alabama, and then packaged it and inspected it. Most of the workers were originally from Puerto Rico and lived in nearby New Haven and New Britain.

But Steven and Bart immediately began to chafe against each other. Bart felt Steven was controlling, and he was suspicious of Bart and his freewheeling style. Bart also had a hard time giving up the role of supervisor. He took to going out on the factory floor every few weeks to make motivational speeches. Bart would call out, "What are we doing here?" There would be an awkward silence.

Someone would say, "We are making QuikClot."

"Yes," Bart would say, "but what are we *really* doing?"

"We are making money," another worker would say.

"NO!" Bart would shout back. "We are saving lives, the lives of people we will never meet and who don't even know we exist. And that is a privilege, a great privilege." Bart hung a sign in the facility that read, "The greatest privilege is to make a difference." The slogan became the official tagline for the company, appearing on its stationery and website. But some of Bart's motivational speeches didn't land quite as well as his talks to his young rowers at Conn College had. Not all the workers seemed to know what to make of Bart and his confusing role and relationship with Steven, and some seemed intimidated by him. They called Bart "Boss Man," "Mr. Bart," or "*El Jefe*," meaning "the chief." But mostly they liked him well enough and were gratified when he intervened on their behalf after learning they used a local check-cashing business, where they were charged a 10 percent fee, instead of depositing their paychecks into a bank. Bart arranged for a representative from the local bank to come to the office and set up checking accounts that paid modest interest for the employees.

During this time Bart took dozens of international trips to

promote QuikClot. In Paris he went to a large international military technology show, where a Russian general approached the QuikClot booth. Through a translator Bart explained the capabilities of the product. Asked if he was interested in QuikClot, the general responded, "No, we don't need that. We have enough soldiers." Bart also flew to Beijing to meet with officials from the Chinese government's equivalent of the FDA, hoping that they might approve QuikClot. The night before the meeting, he and his hosts from the Chinese government went out for a prodigious night of drinking and watching sumo wrestlers. They drank until five in the morning despite the fact that the meeting was scheduled for 9:00 a.m. Bart, already jet-lagged, surmised that the drinking game was a test of his character and fortitude, and he knew he needed to prove his mettle to have any chance of working with the Chinese officials. He was blind drunk at 4:00 a.m., but he staggered to the meeting a few hours later and managed to function. The men he had been drinking with hours earlier seemed remarkably clear eyed. Bart might have passed the drinking test, but the Chinese government declined to move forward with QuikClot.

For all the progress that Bart had made, there was, however, one major problem at the center of QuikClot: it had of course not been selected by the army once the Iraq War had started. And for Bart, this lack of an imprimatur on QuikClot became an obsession. Not only had the army rejected QuikClot, it was, in a letter from the Institute of Surgical Research that Bart had been shown by one of his contacts in the navy, recommending against QuikClot's use. Furthermore, the military's Committee on Tactical Combat Casualty Care, which was dominated by army doctors and tasked with making official policy on trauma medicine, had selected HemCon as the "hemostatic agent of choice." The HemCon company received an initial $400,000 grant from the army, followed by one for $2.45 million. By 2005, HemCon had received $29 million in grants and purchase orders from the army, which was its sole customer. Ultimately its workforce would reach 120 personnel.

Bart hated the way HemCon was being favored and given such significant financial support by the army, especially when the evidence for HemCon's efficacy was often lacking. "HemCon doesn't work," declared the military trauma surgeon Peter Rhee, director of the Navy Trauma Training Center. "I've tried every one of these products, many times, on many different kinds of wounds. I put HemCon on the side of a beating heart once, and it worked great. But for a large, open wound with a lot of bleeding, it's just not effective." As always, the problem with HemCon was not its biochemical method of action, which tended to work beautifully under ideal circumstances, but rather the rigidity of the bandage because it did not conform to jagged, asymmetrical, or deep wounds—which are exactly the kinds of wounds that occur on the battlefield. The theory of the product simply didn't match up to practice. None of these criticisms, however, prevented the army from naming HemCon one of its "Top 10 Greatest Inventions" for 2004, calling it a revolutionary product. This amounted to the army giving itself an award for a product that it had been instrumental in supporting.

Ironically, however, multiple internal army studies, which were not publicly disclosed until 2005, often found that the bandage performed poorly. One study showed that it tended to fall out of the wound after an average of forty-nine minutes, allowing resumed blood flow. Two studies conducted before the start of the Iraq War found that HemCon functioned no better than gauze. In yet another study, only one of ten pigs survived. An army researcher later admitted about HemCon, "It just never lived up to the hype, even in our own laboratories."

Other service branches were deeply skeptical of HemCon, leaving the army its sole backer among US military branches. In remarks to Congress, General William Catto, commanding general of the Marine Corps Systems Command, said, "The Marine Corps does not have any plans to purchase HemCon. The product fails to work in field applications sixty-six [percent] of the time and the product costs $98.00 per bandage." General Catto added, "QuikClot works one hundred percent of the time with zero percent mortality and costs $9.80 per package." The air force and the Coast Guard also rejected HemCon.

Bart would soon realize that the heart of this conflict—in which the army was pitted against everyone else—was an ongoing dispute regarding the amount of heat that zeolite generated when applied to a wound. Here, once again, there was a remarkable divide: the army found one level of heat, while every other party, with one exception, found dramatically lower levels. The differences were extreme and rather puzzling.

All told, five major studies examining the exothermic reaction of QuikClot had been conducted by researchers who were not affiliated with the US Army. In his original trial, Dr. Alam measured temperatures of 42 to 44 degrees Celsius in the tissues immediately surrounding animals' wounds after the application of zeolite. In a follow-up study, he found a range of 51 to 57 degrees Celsius. (By way of reference, 57 degrees Celsius is about 134 degrees Fahrenheit, or just above the typical temperature of hot tap water.) Subsequent researchers at the Uniformed Services University of the Health Sciences found a high temperature of 55 degrees Celsius. Researchers at Zhejiang University in China—who might be the most objective, because presumably they had no skin in the game, being far removed from squabbles within the American military— measured a peak temperature of 45.6 degrees Celsius. The highest temperature was recorded by the Naval Medical Research Center, which found a peak temperature of 70 degrees Celsius, or 158 degrees Fahrenheit, although most of its readings were considerably lower, in the range of 40 to 50 degrees Celsius.

On the other hand, the army, in a 2004 study of zeolite conducted by six scientists from the Institute of Surgical Research, including John Holcomb, reported temperatures that were almost twice as high. Using a different model than Dr. Alam had employed, they inflicted wounds to pigs' livers rather than their femoral arteries and measured a temperature of 100 degrees Celsius—the temperature of boiling water. As part of their investigation, the same scientists conducted an experiment in which they placed ten milliliters of pig blood in a beaker and added ten grams of QuikClot. This is an extremely high ratio of zeolite to liquid. They then stirred the beaker for fifteen minutes and recorded the temperature every minute. In the seventh minute, the mixture reached its peak temperature: 140 degrees Celsius. Strangely, Dr. Alam had done a similar lab experiment and recorded a temperature of only 48 degrees Celsius. When the article about the army's findings was published in the *Journal of Trauma*, it was followed by an unusual letter from a Miami doctor who was neither a military surgeon nor a hematologist. The author compared the use of QuikClot to the barbaric medieval practice of pouring boiling oil on soldiers to cauterize their wounds.

A second study on the heat generated by zeolite came out in 2004, also in the *Journal of Trauma*. This investigation was led by an air force surgeon, even though the air force had already gone on record as endorsing QuikClot. "In practice, burns [produced by QuikClot] were not really a problem that seemed to change the management of the patient," said Lieutenant Colonel Joe Legan, chief surgery consultant to the air force surgeon general. The study was conducted at the air force's Brooks City Base, which is not far from the Institute of Surgical Research. The scientists also used a different model from Alam, one in which pigs were injured in multiple different areas, including the liver, spleen, muscles, veins, arteries, and skin.

Bart was invited to San Antonio to observe the experiment. Bart recalled being aghast when he saw the air force surgeon pour a full packet of QuikClot into the injury site and at times spend as long as thirty minutes before closing the wound. As the researchers wrote later, they "wished to know the wound healing consequences of wound closure with some QuikClot present." When the study was eventually published, it cited temperatures in excess of 95 degrees Celsius in the animal tissues. Significantly, the article never specified with precision how much QuikClot was actually used in the procedures, an unusual omission for a scientific article, in which experimental methods are almost always highly detailed and defined.

When he returned from San Antonio and read the published articles, Bart believed both of the studies had been attempts to get the recorded temperature of QuikClot as high as possible. He also believed that the studies were not based on anything that remotely approximated battlefield conditions. Indeed, a subsequent study of QuikClot as used on the actual battlefield and in a trauma center showed that burns were not a significant issue. The navy surgeon Peter Rhee examined 103 cases of QuikClot use in real-world settings: sixty-nine of these took place on the battlefield in Iraq, and the remainder involved trauma victims at the Los Angeles County+USC Medical Center. While some patients experienced discomfort after the application of QuikClot, there were only three cases of actual burns. Two of those cases healed spontaneously and did not require any medical intervention. Only one patient required aftercare, in this case skin grafting, and took some weeks to heal.

But word of the dangers of QuikClot spread rapidly through the army military community. Bart and members of the Z-Medica staff were now going almost every month to military and medical conferences, where Bart would man a booth, demonstrating both the POGS system and QuikClot and providing samples. QuikClot had been used successfully in Iraq for almost two years now, but he was increasingly encountering army personnel who were affronted by his demonstrations. "You're the people who burn people," he and his staff would be told. "You burn people!" Tim Coakley too would often be at these conferences, acting as a trainer for potential users of QuikClot. Coakley viewed the army medicine elite, whom he saw as under Holcomb's sway, as a kind of single exclusionary unit that moved through the proceedings as if it occupied an entirely different stratum from the other service branches. Coakley called them "the Mogadishu gang." Bart and Coakley sometimes saw Holcomb walking imperiously through the corridors of the hotels where the conventions were typically held, surrounded by obsequious army doctors. At every conference Holcomb would visit the trade show in the exhibit hall, but only briefly. Bart observed that he would tend to stop only at the booths of army-contracted companies and mix it up with the product reps as if they were old friends—which in fact they often were. Many of the men and women working for these companies were former army officers. Holcomb would always walk quickly past the QuikClot booth, never once speaking to Bart or making eye contact with him. It was as if QuikClot did not exist in John Holcomb's world.

Except that it did. In a dramatic demonstration at some of these conferences, Holcomb would place QuikClot into a foam cup of water and watch as the cup melted. In a meeting with the army surgeon general, Holcomb put QuikClot in a cup and poured water onto it until it melted the bottom of the cup. "I don't think we want that on our soldiers," Holcomb said. He would say later that QuikClot reminded him of "John Wayne putting the bowie knife in a candle and sticking it in a wound."

Bart could never figure out why John Holcomb hated QuikClot so much. Bart knew all about Holcomb's valiant service at Mogadishu and had just assumed that Holcomb would do anything possible to save a soldier from bleeding to death. And Bart freely acknowledged that QuikClot had an Achilles' heel, and of course he did not like the idea that even in a very small minority of cases it could cause burns. It bothered him that it would create any kind of discomfort for a patient. Nor did he dispute that if you put copious amounts of QuikClot into water, it could cause boiling. But he also knew that that wasn't relevant to the battlefield unless the medic studiously ignored the product's directions. He knew this in part because in the two years now that QuikClot had been used by the American military, not a single soldier or soldier's family had sued Z-Medica because they believed the product had caused damage. But mainly, as Bart argued to the army people who challenged him, accusing him of harming soldiers, QuikClot had to be viewed in the context of combat and the ongoing and extremely violent war. He would tell the detractors that they had a choice: they could either get a burn or die. Which would they prefer? Bart could never grasp why army medicine couldn't understand that simple calculus, nor could he fathom why, even if the army wanted to stay with HemCon, it couldn't also add QuikClot to its array of products. Why did the army always have to go its own way, and why did it have to destroy the competition?

Army soldiers on the ground in Iraq and Afghanistan agreed. "What's worse, giving your buddy a little burn while you save his life or doing nothing and letting him die?" said Sergeant First Class

Gregory Wilson, an army medic who had trained thousands of soldiers at Fort Dix in New Jersey, in 2005. "Go back, talk to your supply folks, and tell them to get this stuff for you," he told a group of soldiers as they were about to deploy to Iraq and Afghanistan. "And don't let them tell you it's not available. Be aggressive. It can save your life." Another medic said, "It might damage the surrounding tissue, and maybe some surgeon would have to dig it out of me later on, but I'd be alive." Even in a massive wound, medics in the field were not experiencing the heat generated by zeolite. Marine corpsman Seth Secrease was part of a convoy in Iraq in 2005 when a bomb blew up the truck in front of him. He saw the arm of a solider, now almost detached, hanging out of the vehicle ahead. Secrease ran to the soldier in the truck's cabin, applied a tourniquet to his arm, and then poured packets of QuikClot into a profoundly bleeding wound on his hip. Secrease observed the QuikClot resolve the bleeding with its usual remarkable speed, and he did not detect any heat in the pool of blood. The solider survived the immediate blast, but his leg and arm had to be amputated. He lived only another three months, dying at Walter Reed hospital. "But at least he had a chance to say goodbye to his parents," Secrease said. "The tourniquet and the QuikClot allowed him that." Based on stories like that, even though QuikClot had been effectively banned by the army, Joe Dacorta continued to receive calls from army medics asking him to "please send us the QuikClot."

But none of this seemed to get through to the army with its seemingly impenetrable structure. The army remained resolute in its opposition to QuikClot. Bart felt that the army had all the money and all the power while he and Frank had only the truth. Even ever-optimistic Frank grew weary and cynical about the army's conduct. This had become deeply personal for Frank; he fundamentally believed in the essential goodness of American institutions, and his oldest son had been a marine in Desert Storm. Frank believed that the army was not looking out for the common soldier.

Gradually Bart, who had always been a student of history, began to realize that he was unwillingly being pulled into a long and ignoble tradition in the American military. The American military—and the army in particular—had a protracted history of favoring failed products made by military insiders over effective products made by outside innovators who had no political clout. He had been told as much at one of the medical conferences by Bob Harder, a well-respected military contractor who had been supplying first-aid products to the marines for years. Harder said, "If the army didn't invent it, they don't want it. It's been that way for years. But you can change that. You have the best product. Just be patient. Don't go away. Refuse to go away."

There were many stories of good inventions being squelched by the military, but arguably the most infamous examples were the conflict between the Wright brothers and the War Department in the early twentieth century and the debate over the M-16 and AR-15 rifles during the Vietnam War. Between 1900 and 1908, the War Department—now called the Department of Defense— stifled the Wright brothers, even after Orville and Wilbur had successfully flown an airplane. Rather, Washington power brokers backed Samuel Langley, an aviation pioneer and secretary of the Smithsonian Institution as well as a consummate political insider. The War Department and President McKinley gave Langley a $50,000 grant—an enormous sum at the time—to develop his machine, which he called the Aerodrome. Langley's idea was to put a catapult on a houseboat in the middle of the Potomac River that would throw his flying contraption into the air. In the first attempt, in 1903, the wing collided with part of the catapult, leading the Aerodrome to plunge into the river "like a handful of mortar," as one journalist put it. On a second attempt, the rear wing and tail ripped apart. The pilot nearly drowned in the icy Potomac. A member of Congress said, "You tell Langley for me...that the only thing he ever made fly was government money." Langley died three years later after a series of strokes, an old and broken man with nothing to show after eighteen years of work on the project.

Meanwhile, eight days after the pilot in Langley's craft was almost killed, the Wright brothers put a sturdy and elegantly designed craft costing only $1,000 into the air at Kitty Hawk, North Carolina. But even after they had demonstrated they could fly a plane—albeit only for twelve seconds and a distance of 120 feet—the War Department dismissed the Wright brothers and their invention. The two brothers had no political influence. They had not graduated from high school, were from rural Ohio, had failed at a printing business, and had funded their interest in flying with their own bicycle business. They had no scientific training. What they knew, they had mainly acquired from direct pragmatic experience—not unlike Frank Hursey. It would be five years before the War Department awarded the Wright brothers a contract, and even then, the brothers had to force the military's hand. It was only when foreign governments were on the verge of working with the Wright brothers that the United States awarded them a contract.

A similar story of the stifling of innovation played out in the Vietnam War. At the start of the war, the army favored the M-16 rifle—based on a World War II weapon that appeared unsuited for jungle warfare—over a newly developed weapon, the AR-15, created by Eugene Stoner, a small-arms designer who had developed his weapon when working at a tiny gun manufacturer, the ArmaLite Corporation. The M-16 was based on a centuries-old paradigm for guns on the battlefield. Designed for marksmen shooting at targets four hundred to six hundred yards away, it placed a premium on heavy rounds, slow and deliberate fire, and low use of ammunition. It also had a reputation for jamming. Exactly none of these features were what the Vietnam jungle required of a weapon. To survive against the Vietcong, infantrymen needed a light weapon that could shoot light rounds at great speed and at distances of thirty to fifty yards, which is what Stoner's AR-15 was. But the army's so-called Ordnance Corps—a small group of men who decided weapons contracts and had done so for many years—had a cozy relationship with the rifle and munitions makers they were used to working with and refused to buy Stoner's rifle, even when the air force and special forces divisions bought thousands of them and President Kennedy and Secretary of Defense Robert McNamara supported the AR-15. Furthermore, the Ordnance Corps blatantly rigged evidence by by including in the final evaluations "only those tests that will reflect adversely on the AR-15 rifle," as the printed minutes of one of their meetings stated. In Vietnam, the inaccurate, slow, heavy, and uncontrollable M-16 proved no match for the AK-47 used by the Vietcong. Soldiers would put aside several months' salaries in order to buy AR-15s on the black market. American soldiers were killed trying to unjam their M-16 rifles.

Bart began to see himself as just another upstart in a long tradition of upstarts getting crushed by the arrogance of the army. It drove him mad. To Bart, potentially thousands of lives were at stake. Bart had started to think of zeolite in terms of the famous line spoken by Dan Aykroyd and John Belushi in the movie *The Blues Brothers*, in which the actors, playing semideranged bluesmen, repeatedly say they are "on a mission from God" to spread the gospel of their music. Bart too was beginning to believe that he was on a mission from God. He did not think this literally, but the intensity of his desire to deliver on the promise of QuikClot had in fact taken on a religious fervor. The depths of emotion he felt about the product were as powerful as anything that he had ever before experienced outside of the birth of his daughter.

Bart believed that in the lifesaving potential of this simple rock, he had found his mission in life. And now, he knew, he would have to figure out a way to win this war.

In 1985, when Bart was in the Hamptons, he read a best-selling book, *Guerrilla Marketing* by Jay Conrad Levinson. Levinson was the first person to use the term, deriving the idea from guerilla warfare— the methods, common throughout history, whereby untrained or amateur combatants are able to defeat professional armies by using subversive and improvised tactics such as ambushes, sabotage, and deception. In the book Levinson argues that these same concepts should be applied to marketing, which would allow low-budget or disruptive products to penetrate or even overtake established markets. The essence of guerilla marketing lies in its grassroots nature; one doesn't need to reach the masses but rather should attempt to reach a small group of customers with the hope that they will spread the word to a larger audience. Levinson suggested numerous techniques for achieving this goal, such as pop-up retail outlets, "ambient marketing" (advertising in unusual places, such as on the backs of receipts or on posters in locker rooms), and "stealth marketing" (placing a product in a setting in which consumers are unaware it is being advertised, such as in a movie). As Bart looked back on the history of QuikClot, he now realized that he had been so intimidated by the army's power and massive infrastructure that he hadn't thought to use guerrilla marketing techniques to promote the product. But his thinking turned around after a conversation with an army colonel at one of the special operations medical conferences in Tampa, sometime in 2003.

Bart was working the floor at the trade show, as he always did. The colonel came up to talk to him respectfully. This was in itself unusual, as he was used to being either ignored or harassed by army officers. With his weather-beaten face, crew cut, and square jaw, the colonel looked the part of a battle-worn leader. Just about every other word out of his mouth was *fuck*. He said to Bart, "You know, I heard great things about QuikClot. I just want something that works for my soldiers, and I don't give a shit about what lab rats in San Antonio say. That army science is bullshit. My job is to keep soldiers alive."

This moment became an epiphany of sorts for Bart. So far he had received feedback about QuikClot only from the military's professional medical community—attacks from the army, positive reviews from everyone else; he hadn't heard from actual soldiers. Clearly soldiers, the product's ultimate customers, were seeing things differently. Not long after that encounter, Bart met a senior marine corpsman at a training session in Camp Pendleton, the marine base in California. The corpsman said, "QuikClot flat-out works. Don't worry about what the journal articles say. No one reads that stuff. We don't pay any attention to it."

Bart realized that he had been barking up the wrong tree. The upper echelons of army medicine were not the right audience for QuikClot. For QuikClot to break through, he realized that he needed, guerilla-marketing style, to go directly to the consumers. And that meant the soldiers themselves.

But first he would need some help. He hired as an assistant a young woman, Rachel Sancredi, just out of college. Rachel had started only as a temp at On-Site, but Bart saw how eager she was. She was deeply motivated to work on the QuikClot project, perhaps because her father had been a marine in Vietnam, where he had been shot, nonfatally, in the neck. Rachel also had a keen mind, and after Bart hired her full-time, they discussed strategy together. In a meeting with Rachel at a diner, Bart drew a pyramid on a napkin. He divided it into four segments of equal height, like layers in a cake. The top layer he labeled "The Military." On the next layer down, Bart wrote "EMT's and First Responders." On the next section below that, he wrote "Police Officers." Then, on the bottom and widest section of the pyramid, he wrote, "Hospitals."

He said to Rachel that in order for QuikClot to become a breakthrough product on the largest scale, the military, at the top of the pyramid, was the place to start, as Bart had already done. It had the smallest number of decision makers. Furthermore, with the credibility and clout of the military, especially in a time of war, its influence would extend to markets below it on the napkin, eventually all the way down the pyramid to the largest but most complex and difficult-to-reach audience, hospitals. Bart said, "We have been partially successful with the military, but only partially. We are in a conflict with the biggest part of that market, the army. We have to hear directly from the soldiers themselves."

He asked Rachel to create questionnaires for military personnel about their experiences with QuikClot that she could distribute at conferences and training sessions. Rachel soon became a deft and skilled trainer with the product, and the fact that she was young and pretty, as well as very organized and articulate, made her popular among military personnel. She began traveling the country doing sessions on QuikClot, often in tandem with Tim Coakley. Soon Rachel came back with numerous customer testimonials about the product. One was from a medical doctor with the Second Marine Division who had served in Iraq between March and July 2003, who wrote the following on the form that Rachel had created:

> I was the battlefield surgeon for a Marine infantry battalion during the start of OIF [Operation Iraqi Freedom]. I treated ten casualties with [sic] and without a doubt it prevented massive hemorrhage as well as loss of limbs. I recommend wide usage of this product. Outstanding!

Another was from the army's Sergeant David Benoit, who had used the product in Baghdad on May 24, 2003, and who wrote:

> treat a gunshot wound to right thigh...patient was bleeding profussily [sic]. Applied Quickclott [sic]. The bleeding stopped...saving the soldier's leg and life.

This was a great start, Bart said. Bart knew that he had no advertising budget for QuikClot, and Frank would go apoplectic if he requested one. But he now saw he didn't need a budget. Starting in 2003, QuikClot became the subject of an extraordinary amount of publicity, the kind of exposure that most start-ups can only fantasize about. It amounted to a national advertising campaign that cost absolutely nothing.

The flurry began in March 2003 when the *New York Times* wrote about the efficacy of zeolite: "QuikClot converted wounds that were 100 percent fatal into wounds that were 100 percent nonfatal—clots formed and none of the animals died." A similar article, quoting Joe Dacorta and Dr. Alam, appeared in the *Washington Post* a day later. In June, the *Los Angeles Times* published a story, "Lifesaving Product of the War," in which QuikClot is described as "one of the Iraq war's most dramatic lifesaving technologies." The story mentions a marine who was shot in the neck. The bullet nicked the carotid artery before exiting from the back of his skull. The journalist wrote, "QuikClot was poured onto his wound, sealing it immediately," and concluded that the marine was "a casualty that probably would have been a fatality in the Persian Gulf war." *The Early Show* on CBS noted how QuikClot induces "rapid coagulation of wounds." The *Economist* stated the product "stems even severe arterial bleeding." Other positive notices appeared in *Businessweek*, the *Wall Street Journal*, Fox News, *Outdoor Life*, *Popular Science*, and the military publication *Stars and Stripes*. Even Frank finally got some publicity for being an inventor. In its November 2003 issue, *Scientific American* named Francis X. Hursey among its top 50 "research leaders of the year." Remarkably, this would be the only recognition from the national scientific community that Frank ever received.

In April 2004 the nationally syndicated comic strip *Doonesbury* featured QuikClot when one of its main characters, B.D., an army lieutenant, is blasted by a rocket grenade in Iraq. His medic calls for a helicopter and applies QuikClot. B.D. is medevaced and then operated on in the combat hospital. Given the severity of the injury, the medic is shocked that B.D. even survives. Frank and Bart were in the office on a Tuesday morning when they got a call from a friend telling them that QuikClot had appeared in the strip. They immediately arranged for a shipment of QuikClot to be sent to Garry Trudeau, *Doonesbury*'s creator, who lived nearby in Connecticut. Much later, QuikClot was featured in the movie *Shooter*, starring Mark Wahlberg. Early on in the film, Wahlberg's character, Bob Lee Swagger, is shot multiple times. He finds a packet of QuikClot in a stolen medical supply bag, rips open the packet with his teeth, and empties its contents into the bullet hole in his shoulder. He then pours a heaping pile of it into a second wound around his waist, grimacing. Even though the wounds appear to have been life threatening, Swagger quickly recovers and goes on to kill his assailants and many other people by the end of the movie. *Shooter* was a massive box office hit, and its portrayal of QuikClot raised the profile of the product. This proved to be gratifying but also a mixed blessing, as the movie melodramatically depicted the pain generated by application of the product.

Bart and Rachel placed the accolades for QuikClot on the Z-Medica website. At the same time Bart and Frank, in conjunction with Joe Dacorta, undertook a campaign to attempt to reduce the heat generated by zeolite as well as looking at less messy ways to deliver the product. They experimented with putting the granules of zeolite into what amounted to a tea bag, a porous fabric pouch with four compartments, which the FDA approved. With Joe Dacorta and the Office of Naval Research acting as a funder and intermediary, Bart and Frank also began working with a University of California mineral scientist, Galen Stucky. In his lab Stucky studied the fundamental mechanism of action that caused zeolite to work. He and his team discovered that in addition to zeolite absorbing the water in blood, which left the clotting factors, zeolite's positively charged calcium ions also facilitated the clotting cascade, just as Tim Coakley had suspected. But the calcium also created heat in reaction to the water molecules in blood. Stucky and his graduate students experimented with replacing the calcium in zeolite with silver, which also contains positive ions, with the hope that it might reduce the heat reaction. Unfortunately, soaking zeolite in silver didn't much reduce the heat, but it did have the benefit of providing antibacterial properties, reducing the risk of infections. Bart and Frank, now working with some research scientists of their own employed at Z-Medica, applied for and received FDA approval for a new silver version of QuikClot.

But there still of course remained the issue of actually getting the army to purchase QuikClot. Here too Bart and Rachel discovered that the army wasn't quite as impenetrable and monolithic as it appeared. In talking to Joe Dacorta, they learned that the most senior medical officers within individual army divisions had what were called impact cards—essentially credit cards they could use independently to make purchases deemed mission critical. At conferences, and even just by cold-calling them, Bart and Rachel began reaching out to divisional surgeons at various army bases. They found most of the doctors open and approachable.

The first to bite, early in 2003, was the Third Infantry Division out of Fort Stewart, Georgia, a legendary outfit that had served under George Patton in World War II. The division well needed the approximately $100,000 it spent on QuikClot: in April 2003 the entire division crossed the deserts of Iraq in less than three days. Next came a sizable order from the First Infantry Division, popularly known as "the Big Red One," in Fort Riley, Kansas, which was comprised of tens of thousands of soldiers and had been in continuous operation longer than any other army division. That was followed by an order from the Tenth Mountain Division, an infantry outfit in Fort Drum, New York, and finally one from doctors at the army's 101st Airborne Division in Fort Campbell, Kentucky.

Bart realized that the grizzled colonel who had spoken to him at the special operations conference had been right: soldiers didn't "give a shit" what the lab rats in San Antonio said.

And certainly a solider named Ryan Kules did not. On November 24, 2005, Lieutenant Kules of the army's First Armored Division had Thanksgiving dinner with the twenty-four soldiers under his command at his base near Taji, just north of Baghdad. That dinner was the last thing Kules would remember for weeks. At that point he had been in Iraq for nine months, leading patrols, raids, and searches, trying among other things to find hidden IEDs. Kules had grown up in Scottsdale, Arizona, and graduated from Arizona State University. He'd joined the army because he wanted to give back to his country and be part of something larger than himself.

Five days after the Thanksgiving dinner, on November 29, Kules's patrol was on the way back from an early-morning mission to search a house where military intelligence believed there was a weapon or explosive of some kind. As the senior officer in the command, Kules had chosen to ride in the lead Humvee even though he didn't have to. "I rode in the lead because part of being a leader is putting yourself out in front," he said later. His vehicle ran over four artillery shells buried in the road. Two soldiers inside the vehicle with Kules were immediately killed. Kules was thrown about a hundred feet from the Humvee and landed in a wadi, a small irrigation creek. It took the medics ten minutes to find him. When they did, Kules was still strapped into the seat of his vehicle but trying to stand up. His left leg and right arm had been blown off. Medics put a tourniquet on his left arm, which was also severely damaged, and QuikClot into the stump that remained of his left leg. As usual, the bleeding was controlled. A helicopter arrived, landing on the narrow road, and took Kules to the combat hospital in Baghdad. Kules lost his pulse more than once and could have been pronounced technically dead on two occasions. Later medics found his right arm and left leg in the dirt.

Kules's wife, a kindergarten teacher in Arizona, was notified about her husband's status at the end of the school day. Kules was flown to Germany and finally the United States. When his parents and wife first saw him in the hospital, he was almost entirely wrapped in bandages. The only visible parts of him were his forehead, a toe, and his ears, caked with dried blood. Kules underwent three dozen surgeries and remained an inpatient at Walter Reed for four months.

Kules lost his wedding ring during the blast. It was found later, now warped and oval shaped, near the bomb site. Kules had it repaired so he could wear it once again. He is now the father of three teenage children and a senior officer at the national headquarters of the Wounded Warrior Project. In 2020, federal legislation to boost funding for adaptive technologies in housing for wounded veterans, named in his honor, was signed by the president.

During all of this, Ryan Kules never knew that the QuikClot given to him by the medic, which had probably saved his life, had been administered against official army protocol.

Stories like this, and his belief that adequate care was being denied soldiers, made Bart increasingly feel as if he was going to crack and that his mission from God was being stifled. Sometime late in 2005, Bart picked up the phone in his office in Connecticut and dialed a Texas number.

"May I speak to Colonel Holcomb, please?"

"How can I help you?" Holcomb said after Bart eventually got through to him. Bart tried not to let his voice shake from either fear or anger.

"Well, as you know, our product has been adopted by the other service branches and is having good success. I am of course aware that the army has chosen to go with other products." There was silence on the other end of the line.

"Well," Bart persevered, "I was wondering if we might possibly join forces. As you know, our product has the backing of the other three branches of the military. I don't see why the army needs to be an outlier." More silence. Then laughter. "I just don't see why QuikClot can't be added to the existing products that the army is using," Bart said. More laughter.

"Yeah, sure...of course," Holcomb said, his voice dripping with sarcasm.

That was the first and last time John Holcomb and Bart Gullong ever spoke.

By this time, Holcomb appeared not to be that interested in QuikClot anymore. By 2005, John Holcomb had moved on to something else—a drug to stop traumatic bleeding so powerful that it made QuikClot and HemCon seem like child's play.

It was a drug called Factor Seven.

CHAPTER EIGHT

The Danger of Using a
Sledgehammer to Crack a Nut

AROUND SIX MONTHS after Bart impetuously and unsuccessfully called Holcomb, at 12:30 p.m. on May 4, 2006, a United States Army private, Caleb Lufkin, age twenty-four, was flown by helicopter into the compound of the Tenth Combat Support Hospital in downtown Baghdad. The combat hospital was housed inside the Ibn Sina Hospital, which during Saddam Hussein's rule had provided medical care to high-ranking Iraqi officials. The facility was in the so-called International Zone, a heavily guarded area encircled by concrete walls and razor wire that had once been home to many Iraqi government offices—including the parliament building and the palaces of Saddam Hussein—as well as the US embassy. Lufkin was lifted out of the helicopter and placed in a jeep that carried him the hundred yards across the makeshift airfield to the receiving area of the hospital. Immediately a team of doctors and nurses began furiously tending to him. Lufkin was weak and bloody, but his body, except for his arm, appeared largely intact.

A little more than half an hour earlier, Lufkin had been riding in a heavily armored truck in downtown Baghdad. He and his crew had the exquisitely nerve-racking task of removing roadside bombs from the streets of the city. But Lufkin had told his parents they should not worry because his vehicle was so well protected that the bombs couldn't penetrate the armor. This perhaps unrealistic optimism seemed characteristic of Lufkin, who appeared to be the quintessential all-American kid. He was from Knoxville, Illinois, was tall and strapping, and had been a baseball star in high school. During his senior year, he'd hit the home run that won Knoxville High School the conference title. He also played the banjo, fished, hunted, and rode motorcycles. While attending Illinois Central College, Lufkin had earned his firefighting certification, and then he'd volunteered for the East Galesburg and Knoxville fire departments. He'd also worked with his father in the family concrete and construction business.

Just before noon on May 4, the last thing that Lufkin saw before the improvised explosive device went off under the truck was a boy riding a bicycle. The device that detonated under him was a military-grade bomb, more powerful than usual, and capable of penetrating armor. Two soldiers riding with Lufkin were killed instantly. Somehow a medic managed to pull Lufkin from the vehicle through the gunner's hatch. As the truck became engulfed in flames, medics attended to Lufkin, applying tourniquets to his arms and legs. Iraqi civilians crowded around him in the roadway.

Caleb Lufkin's arrival at the combat hospital was captured by a CNN camera crew that later made a documentary, aired on the network, called *Combat Hospital*. The scene was also observed by Robert Little, a war reporter for the *Baltimore Sun*, who published stories in that paper about his experiences in the combat hospital later that year. When Lufkin arrived at the triage room at the Tenth

Combat Support Hospital, the surgeon, David Steinbruner, said to him, "Holy crap…OK, bud. All right, clean him off, guys. What's your name?"

Lufkin said, "Caleb."

"All right, Caleb…Breathe deep for me, Caleb." The nurses removed his boot, revealing a bloody sock. There appeared to be fractures in his leg. His ankle was shattered, and his kneecap so damaged that it had turned into what the doctors called bone dust. His right hand, which was covered with blood and grime, was barely attached to the rest of his arm. Where his wrist should have been was merely a bit of flesh and skin. The team sedated him and prepared to give him a breathing tube.

Lufkin asked Steinbruner, "Am I fucking dying?"

Steinbruner said, "You having trouble breathing there?"

"A little bit," Lufkin said.

"Can you move that hand at all?"

Lufkin lifted his hand slightly. "Yeah. Good. That's a good sign, bud," Steinbruner said. The nurses and technicians were crowding around. One of them shouted out a blood pressure reading.

"Hey. Am I going to lose my fucking leg?"

"I don't know. That I don't know…We'll try to save it if we can, OK?"

"Try," Lufkin said.

"Don't you dare try and die on me, OK? I didn't give you permission," Steinbruner said.

"Don't let me die," Lufkin pleaded.

"I won't let you die. I promise."

"Promise?" asked Lufkin.

"I promise. I give you my word."

Lufkin didn't cry out once during the entire exchange.

In the back of the small room where Lufkin was being treated,

John Holcomb, wearing green scrubs, observed the team, occa-sionally offering advice and giving instructions. This was common practice for Holcomb, who often visited war zones. As commander of the Institute of Surgical Research, he largely had carte blanche to go in and out of Iraq and Afghanistan as he chose.

Sometime after Lufkin arrived, John Holcomb called for Lufkin to be injected with a new and controversial drug called Factor Seven. After the injection Lufkin was brought into surgery, where Holcomb was the surgeon who operated on his left leg. His doctors commented that his bleeding had slowed remarkably, a turnaround they attributed to the administration of the Factor Seven. "His blood pressure was eighty, he'd lost about forty percent of his blood volume, and in surgery an hour later he's stable and hardly bleed-ing at all," Holcomb later said in an interview. "We're learning how to deal with these massive injuries."

The drug given to Caleb Lufkin—technically termed Recombi-nant Factor VIIa, but more frequently called simply Factor Seven A or just Factor Seven for short—was an extraordinary departure from every previous entrant in the race to stop catastrophic bleed-ing. All the preceding hemostatic agents that had been deployed on battlefields—the doomed Red Cross fibrin bandage, HemCon, and QuikClot—were topical agents applied externally in the form of bandages or granular powders and therefore were classified simply as "medical devices." But Factor Seven was a drug—a power-ful and expensive drug—administered intravenously that worked systemically throughout the body and managed bleeding that was not treatable by external interventions like tourniquets and dress-ings. Factor Seven was produced by Denmark's Novo Nordisk, one of the largest pharmaceutical companies in the world.

The injection administered to Caleb Lufkin was given on an "off-label" basis—that is, for a use outside of the ones for which the drug was approved. Factor Seven had been approved by the FDA in 1999, but solely as a treatment for hemophilia. Hemophilia, a serious blood clotting disorder, is an extremely rare condition: only about 400,000 people globally suffer from the disease. People diagnosed with hemophilia have low levels of two of the body's clotting factors, either Factor Eight or Factor Nine, which causes the clotting cascade to be interrupted midstream. Without treatment, a person with the illness can bleed for days after a procedure as simple as a tooth extraction. Even biting one's tongue can send a patient to the hospital. In the past people with hemophilia bled to death before reaching adulthood. Factor Seven worked by increasing the amount of the seventh factor of the body's clotting system as much as a thousandfold, thereby jump-starting the clotting cascade and compensating for the missing eighth or ninth factors. Producing the drug was extremely complicated, taking up to a year, which meant it was remarkably expensive. Factor Seven, at $5,000 or more a dose, was one of the costliest drugs in the world.

From the very beginning, the use of Factor Seven for conditions other than hemophilia had been controversial. The drug had an adequate safety profile when used for patients with hemophilia, but there were concerns about what would occur when its use was extended further, particularly after John Holcomb became the drug's champion—its Johnny Appleseed—for Factor Seven's use on army soldiers. The essential question was: For those without a hereditary clotting disorder, would the drug be *too* good at clotting blood? When given to soldiers like Caleb Lufkin, would Factor Seven create clots not only at the wound site but also in the wrong places—in the heart and lungs and brain—where they could cause heart attacks and strokes and potentially kill people? Or, more pointedly, with Factor Seven, had the army now gone too far in its zeal to stop traumatic bleeding? Had Holcomb's desire to save lives, honorably born from the trauma of Mogadishu, led to desperate measures?

These would prove difficult questions to answer, but one fact would soon become clear. Three weeks after receiving Factor Seven during his operation in Baghdad, Caleb Lufkin died of cardiac arrest.

In 1999, seven years before Lufkin died, around the time that Frank Hursey and Bart Gullong met for the first time at Paradise Pizza and six years after the Battle of Mogadishu, John Holcomb flew to Israel with other trauma specialists from the American military to meet with their counterparts in the Israeli army. There he met Uri Martinowitz, a bearded, bespectacled hematologist and trauma adviser to the Israeli army and a retired lieutenant colonel. Martinowitz was about ten years Holcomb's senior, but they shared a common traumatic experience. Soon after he graduated from medical school in 1973, Martinowitz had treated waves of casualties in the Yom Kippur War, just as Holcomb had done in Mogadishu. Martinowitz said, "The worst feeling in a physician's life is when you are just standing there, with nothing you can do while your patient dies. I never wanted to be that helpless again." Holcomb and Martinowitz surely bonded over losing patients who had bled to death, and they left the conference agreeing that a newly introduced drug, Factor Seven, had great potential to be the next candidate in the race to stop bleeding.

The development of Factor Seven was the single obsession of a Swedish doctor, Ulla Hedner, who had begun her quest in 1959 at age twenty. A lean, striking-looking woman with a shock of reddish-blond hair, Hedner worked as an unpaid lab technician in the General Hospital in Malmö before she received her medical degree. The lab focused on the study of blood coagulation, and it was there that Hedner first became fascinated by blood and its disorders. Hedner also worked on the hemophilia unit. As she wrote later:

> The hemophiliacs who were inpatients at the medical clinic...spent a lot of time in the basement where the laboratory was situated if they were well enough to move around. Like the rest of the staff, I got to know these hemophilia boys extremely well....A strong family bond and family feeling developed between patients and staff.

In an interview, Hedner said:

> It was so clear that the patients with hemophilia...were so lousily treated. I had to apologize to these families that we were so lousy in treating them....And then I had this stubbornness—I don't want to give up. So I thought—it should be possible to find something for those patients that could induce hemostasis without side effects.

Hedner, like Uri Martinowitz and John Holcomb after her, had experienced the powerlessness of seeing a patient bleed to death in front of her. As she wrote, "This tragic event occurred...when I was working as laboratory technician at the hospital in Malmö. I was sent to take a blood sample from the patient in question, a woman who had given birth to her first child. An overwhelming feeling of helplessness characterized the whole situation, when the blood, completely lacking any tendency to coagulate, just ran out of her until she died."

Just like John Holcomb, Hedner set out on an obsessive quest to stop bleeding. Hedner became fascinated by a subset of hemophilia patients, those with what are called inhibitors. Most people with hemophilia can manage their condition by receiving injections of concentrates of the factors they lack. However, a small subset of patients, perhaps 10 percent, have inhibitors that cause the body to reject treatment. These patients are twice as likely to be hospitalized and are at increased risk of death.

Normal clotting is initiated by a substance called tissue factor found in the inner layers of the blood vessel walls. Upon an injury to the wall, tissue factor is exposed to circulating blood, at which point it forms a tight complex with Factor Seven, which in turn leads to the formation of a clot. Over many lonely hours in the lab, Hedner discovered that an injection of vast amounts of Factor Seven into tissue factor led directly to the activation of Factor Ten. In other words, Factors Eight and Nine could be completely bypassed and the patient would still be able to form a clot. It was as if the drug allowed its recipients to advance three steps on a board game rather than one. In this way it no longer mattered that patients with inhibitors didn't respond to treatments of additional amounts of Factor Eight and Nine. With Hedner's drug, they no longer needed to. She had found a way to save them.

Between 1978 and 1981, Hedner harvested pure Factor Seven from human plasma. She first used her plasma-derived Factor Seven on a patient with hemophilia in 1981. The patient had a muscle bleed, which for someone with hemophilia can be fatal. Upon receiving Factor Seven, the patient recovered more quickly than expected. Next Hedner treated an eleven-year-old boy, Johann, after he lost a tooth. The boy's family was concerned that he would bleed for days. Riding a night train, Hedner arrived in the boy's town at five in the morning. She injected Factor Seven and watched as a clot formed on the boy's gums.

Having proven that her drug worked, Hedner needed to partner with a pharmaceutical company to produce the drug at scale. The natural fit was Novo Nordisk, which is based in Denmark but has a large presence in Sweden. The original company, Nordisk Insulinlaboratorium, was established in 1923. From its inception Nordisk produced insulin, for which it is still famous; today Novo Nordisk produces half of the world's insulin supply. But over the decades Novo Nordisk expanded into chronic diseases more generally, which made it a good landing place for Ulla Hedner.

Hedner arrived at Novo Nordisk as a research scientist in 1983, only to find that the marketing department was deeply skeptical about her work. Its reluctance to embrace the drug was understandable because at the time there were only six hemophilia patients with inhibitors in all of Sweden. But as always, Hedner was relentless, and in 1985 she received the green light to develop Factor Seven as a drug. Unlike the human plasma–derived Factor Seven she had created earlier, she would help develop at Novo Nordisk a "recombinant" product—that is, one generated entirely in the lab by virtue of newly emerging DNA technology that combined genetic material from multiple sources. The recombinant version of Factor Seven would be much purer and remove the risk of infecting patients with diseases like HIV that could be carried in the human plasma.

But creating a drug through recombinant technology was exquisitely arduous. It required first that the gene for human Factor Seven be cloned and introduced into the kidney cells of baby hamsters. Then those cells needed to be cultured in a fluid made up of newborn calf serum. Then followed a prolonged purification process to remove any viruses carried by the animals. After all the trouble and expense involved, one would think the drug would look more impressive—but it was simply a clear liquid that appeared no different from water.

To offset the costs, Novo Nordisk took advantage of the Orphan Drug Act, an arrangement adopted by many countries to help pharmaceutical companies bear the cost of creating critical drugs for rare diseases and small patient groups. Factor Seven, of course, was the very definition of an orphan drug. Hedner heard of the Orphan Drug Act only by pure happenstance when she sat next to a New York health-care attorney who told her about the program on a flight from Sweden to the United States. Orphan drug programs are created with the goal of benefiting the public, but critics have long charged that drug companies exploit the loopholes within these policies, such as softer restrictions, extended patent protection lengths, and tax breaks. There have been numerous cases in which an orphan drug, originally thought to serve only a small number of patients, took off, through off-label prescribing, to become a "blockbuster" drug—defined as one that nets more than $1 billion annually in sales. Remarkably, seven of the ten best-selling drugs in the United States in 2015 originated as orphan drugs, including the drug Humira, primarily used for arthritis, which saw more than $8 billion in sales. In these cases, the pharmaceutical company enjoys the best of both worlds—the unique advantages and support to develop an obscure drug followed by the profits of a mass-market drug. But even with the assistance of the Orphan Drug Act, it would take Novo Nordisk a total of ten and a half years to bring Factor Seven to the market.

Even though it appeared destined to be an obscure drug, from the beginning there was always something different about Factor Seven—something uniquely tantalizing. What hematologists and surgeons eventually realized was that Hedner had altered, at least conceptually, the entire paradigm of how medical doctors viewed catastrophic bleeding. This is how Richard Dutton, a trauma anesthesiologist, put it in 2011:

> Now, another thing about Factor Seven, it provoked a whole school of thinking. Prior to the year 2000, we didn't think we could control coagulation from outside. So the analogy I use for the anesthesiologists I talk to is, for forty years, if the surgeon says, "Could you make this person stop moving," we can pick up a syringe, give them a drug, and they become paralyzed. We can reverse that effect very cleanly when we want it reversed, and you don't really regard this as a miracle but in some way it is. It is very unusual that we have that degree of control. The advent of Factor Seven put the thought in our heads that we could do the same thing for the coagulation system—that we could turn it on and off in a discrete fashion.

In other words, Ulla Hedner almost singlehandedly found a way to turn clotting on and off. This must have been a dream come true for doctors like John Holcomb and Uri Martinowitz who had experienced the agony of having patients bleed to death in their hands. The idea that one could potentially stop that bleeding with an injection was extremely seductive, and indeed it would be that very allure that would ultimately lead to Factor Seven's downfall.

A month after the meeting of Israeli and American military doctors in the spring of 1999, Uri Martinowitz used Factor Seven on a wounded soldier in Israel. The patient was a nineteen-year-old who had been shot in the stomach at point-blank range and brought into the Sheba Medical Center on the brink of death. At the time of the incident, Martinowitz was planning to conduct a trial of Factor Seven on pigs before he used the drug on humans, but he chose that night not to wait any longer to do the study. Martinowitz called for an injection of Factor Seven. The soldier's bleeding largely stopped within ten minutes, and he survived.

Martinowitz and his colleagues published the case report of the miraculous save in the British medical journal the *Lancet*. Published only five months after the incident, the article does not read like a typical medical journal article. It reads like a short story. One can feel the unabashed excitement about the drug come through in the writing. Martinowitz and colleagues describe vividly "a desperate attempt to control the bleeding," adding that "a fatal outcome seemed inevitable," but that "the oozing stopped immediately."

Ian Roberts, an English doctor who would go on to become one of the world's leading experts on traumatic bleeding, remembers reading the article when it first appeared. He was appalled by it and believed the *Lancet* should never have published the piece. For Roberts, the story of the soldier went against the established rules of medical evidence. He considered the incident to be simply an anecdote, a study of exactly one person—which in his view was the diametric opposite of a randomized clinical trial, the gold standard of evidence-based medicine, which involves hundreds or thousands of participants. A clinical trial compares two groups, one of whom receives a drug or treatment while the other one does not. The two groups are matched as closely as possible in all other respects so that the only significant difference between them is the use of the drug or treatment, a process that largely eliminates bias from the results. To Roberts, anecdotal evidence such as Martinowitz's case study was highly misleading, if not destructive. He said, "Things get into medicine by the back door this way. Anecdotes about success pile up, and, before you know it, it's the standard treatment, but it's still not proven." But if Martinowitz wanted to make a splash, he had

chosen the right outlet to disseminate his story. The *Lancet* is arguably the world's leading medical journal, with an impact factor—
a measure of the number of times the journal's articles are cited by
other scholars—greater even than that of the august *New England
Journal of Medicine*. Even Roberts admitted that the article was brilliantly effective. "It was visual, compelling. It impacted the heart
more than it did the mind, the emotions rather than the intellect.
Certainly it was great marketing for Novo Nordisk," he said.

Word of Martinowitz's dramatic save ran like a depth charge
through the relatively small world of trauma surgeons and hema-
tologists, who are unaccustomed to good news. Within the United
States Army, understandably, interest ran especially high. Robert
Vandre, director of the army's Combat Casualty Care Research
Program in Fort Detrick, Maryland, said the treatment could be
widely used. "It's got incredible potential," Vandre said. In March
of 2001, John Holcomb and trauma doctors from around the
United States gathered in Chicago. The meeting was sponsored by
Novo Nordisk, and the purpose was to discuss staging a large-scale
randomized clinical trial to study the efficacy of Factor Seven on
human patients suffering from trauma. But the FDA prevented the
proposed trial, stating there was not sufficient evidence the drug
was safe for testing on people. Actually, because of the degree of
its concern, the FDA blocked all human testing of Factor Seven in
the United States. This forced Novo Nordisk to conduct the trial
outside of the United States.

Finally, a surgeon at a hospital in South Africa agreed to
coordinate the study in 2002. What became known as the Boffard
study examined the impact of Factor Seven on the two predominant types of physical trauma: blunt and penetrating. Blunt trauma,
which is what would typically occur in a car accident, affects the
whole system, while penetrating trauma involves specific damage to

a localized area, such as that caused by a knife or gunshot wound. The hypothesis of the Boffard study was simple: that the group randomized to the Factor Seven condition would require fewer blood transfusions because the drug would stem blood loss. The study also tracked serious adverse events such as heart attacks and strokes, which are termed thromboembolic events. *Thrombo-* refers to clotting, while *emboli* are pieces of clot that detach and drift off, blocking important blood vessels in other parts of the body.

The results of the study were published in the *Journal of Trauma* and appeared to report positive outcomes. The investigators observed a significant reduction in blood transfusion after Factor Seven administration to blunt trauma patients, and what they described as a "trend" toward reduced transfusion for those with penetrating trauma. The study also found very similar rates of thromboembolic events between the control and treatment groups. But the results were immediately criticized. Boffard had omitted from his final results a specific group of patients—those who had died within forty-eight hours of injury. The removal of those patients made the overall outcome look favorable, but when those patients were put back into the study, there appeared to be no statistically significant difference between those who were treated with Factor Seven and those who were not.

Hematologists Kathryn Webert and Morris Blajchman of McMaster University in Canada accused the researchers of "information laundering." They wrote in a letter to the *Journal of Trauma*:

> The results of this important study, based on the data relevant to the clearly stated primary outcome, are negative....Yet the authors of the study suggest that it is a positive study....The reader cannot help but wonder

whether undue influence from the sponsor was put on the investigators to report the findings in a positive light to better serve the sponsor's marketing objectives.

Nonetheless, John Holcomb, who received the early results of the Boffard study, believed they justified the US Army moving forward with Factor Seven in the field. Just as he had done previously with HemCon and the fibrin bandage, Holcomb would become an unabashed advocate of Factor Seven. "When it works, it's amazing," he was quoted as saying in 2006, using the same adjective—*amazing*— that he had used to describe HemCon. Of course, using Factor Seven for conditions other than hemophilia was not approved by the FDA, but this in itself was not a problem; many drugs are used outside of their approved uses based on a doctor's discretion. And as commander of the Institute of Surgical Research, Holcomb essentially had carte blanche to greenlight Factor Seven's use on army soldiers. The way the rather opaque institution had been set up, John Holcomb was quite literally a commander, one who could dictate policy. As a doctor who worked under Holcomb, and who would later challenge the army's use of Factor Seven in a whistleblower lawsuit, said about John Holcomb and the Institute of Surgical Research: "The ISR is unique in that the person who was in charge of the trauma database, the commander of the institute who is in charge of research and the person who is in charge of clinical practice guidelines, was all the same person. And the person who was the commander and was responsible for evaluations was all the same person."

The arrangement between Novo Nordisk and the army was perhaps made easier because they were already extremely well acquainted with each other. A significant part of the American military budget is spent on pharmaceutical drugs—in 2002 that number was $3 billion, and by 2011 it was almost $7 billion. Much of this expenditure is for older, retired veterans, many of whom require insulin for diabetes, much of which is manufactured by Novo Nordisk. And it was to Novo Nordisk's great advantage to "get in" with the army, particularly for an emerging and controversial drug like Factor Seven. It is well known in pharmaceutical circles that adoption by the military carries special prestige, as well as pragmatic value, for individual drugs. When medications are added to the military's Central Command formulary, they become available to all military hospitals and pharmacies. It is assumed that military doctors will continue to prescribe the medications they used in the military when they return to civilian medicine.

John Holcomb formally made the decision to move forward with Factor Seven as a standard treatment for bleeding soldiers in Iraq in February 2004, and he was supported in this by army leadership. Around this time, Holcomb also approached Joe Dacorta and Mike Given at the Office of Naval Research to see if the navy and marines would adopt the drug too, just as he had earlier approached them about HemCon. Given and Dacorta consulted with each other, as well as with Dr. Alam, and as a group rejected Factor Seven. The navy and marines were satisfied with QuikClot and did not see any reason to take on the risks that Factor Seven entailed. Given had also heard from Israeli combat doctors who had been unimpressed by the drug's performance.

The drug arrived at army combat hospitals shortly thereafter, in early 2004. The army's guidelines were liberal, allowing doctors to inject the drug before it was clear that patients were suffering life-threatening hemorrhage. By 2006, as a journalist who was on the ground in combat hospitals in Iraq wrote, "Army protocol in Baghdad called for injecting it into virtually every casualty with signs of serious bleeding."

Back in Connecticut, Bart Gullong and Frank Hursey knew absolutely nothing about Factor Seven until Joe Dacorta mentioned to them that John Holcomb had adopted the drug. Bart was flabbergasted when he heard about the army's latest pursuit. It seemed desperate to him. As far as he had known, the army had invested resources into HemCon. As Bart processed the news, he thought, *My gosh, Holcomb will do anything not to adopt QuikClot.* Even imperturbable Frank was distressed; as he learned more about the use of Factor Seven in Iraq and Afghanistan, he would come to think that its use was deeply irresponsible in nature.

Indeed, after the army rolled out Factor Seven, a chorus of hematologists and regulators sounded the alarm about the risk that it would cause unwanted clotting. "When you give a patient a powerful clot-promoting medication, you may well induce a clot some place you don't want one," said Rodger Bick, an eminent University of Texas hematologist. Jawed Fareed, a pharmacologist and director of the hemostasis and thrombosis research program at Loyola University Chicago Stritch School of Medicine, said, "The moment [Factor Seven] reaches the bloodstream, it triggers clotting. It's a completely irresponsible and inappropriate use of a very, very dangerous drug."

Furthermore, there was a conceptual problem concerning Factor Seven that led some doctors to question how useful and safe the drug was for trauma patients. Dr. Alam put it this way: "The coagulation cascade has thirteen separate proteins that have to get activated sequentially to generate a clot. If one factor is missing and you replenish it, a clot can be generated. However, in trauma patients often all of the factors are extremely low and many are barely measurable. Thus, even if you provide *supra* normal levels of just one factor, the cascade will not flow normally to generate a clot. Giving additional plasma or red blood cells can overcome the deficit much better than Factor Seven, as those transfusions can supply many missing factors. In fact, plasma can supply almost all the factors." Dr. Stephan Mayer, a professor of neurology and neurosurgery at New York Medical College, added that soldiers exposed to Factor Seven after being wounded by IEDs were at particular risk of complications. "The violence of these explosives creates vulnerabilities in the veins and arteries throughout the body, mini-ruptures if you will. When Factor Seven is injected, it goes everywhere in the bloodstream. It can go to brains or lungs— wherever there has been damage in the bloodstream—and try and create clots. In this way trauma victims are at particular risk."

Those who voiced such concerns would prove to be prescient. Military doctors started seeing unusual complications in soldiers after Factor Seven was introduced in the war on terror. As reported by the doctor and best-selling author Atul Gawande in the *New England Journal of Medicine* in late 2004, military surgeons observed "startling" rates of blood clots in the lungs and veins of soldiers who had undergone operations. Initial data at that time showed that 5 percent of soldiers treated with Factor Seven at the military's flag-ship Walter Reed hospital developed lung clots, which resulted in two deaths. At Landstuhl Regional Medical Center in Germany— the largest American military hospital outside the continental United States—doctors reported that they had observed unusual clots in the hearts and arteries of young soldiers that resembled those typically seen in older patients. "We see some strokes," said Lieutenant Colonel Warren Dorlac, director of trauma surgery and critical care at Landstuhl, in 2006. Dr. Walter Dzik of Massachusetts General Hospital said, "It is not that we just don't know what the right thing to do is, but I would say that we do know that when you use [Factor Seven] outside of its approved uses it is accompanied by these [side effects] which can be fatal." Rodger

159

Bick was more blunt. "It's insane, using it that way. Absolutely insane," he said.

Major publications and medical journals sounded the alarm. After Ian Roberts, the English doctor and bleeding expert who was head of the World Health Organization's Collaborating Centre on Research and Training in Injury Control, read the *Lancet* article, he investigated the use of Factor Seven and wrote to the British secretary of state for defence questioning the drug's use without evidence of safety. (The British army also experimented with Factor Seven, although on a much smaller scale than the Americans.) The *British Medical Journal* then ran a story titled "British Soldiers Are 'Guinea Pigs' for New Use of Blood Clotting Agent." The *New York Times*, in its profile of Holcomb—entitled "Army's Aggressive Surgeon Is Too Aggressive for Some"—cited critics who said that "his efforts, however well intended, may be doing more harm than good." Years later, doctors from the University of Padua in Italy wrote an article about Factor Seven for the medical journal *Artificial Organs*. The authors called for guidelines specifying the drug was to be used extremely judiciously and conservatively, and only in the sickest of patients. They concluded their article with these words: "In managing bleeding, we must not use a sledgehammer to crack a nut."

At the heart of all the outcry was one fundamental question: Was the drug simply too powerful? Was using it equivalent to using a sledgehammer to crack a nut? Could it kill soldiers? Louis Aledort, an eminent hematologist at Mount Sinai Hospital, had a direct answer: "Of course some of them are dying from it.... If you give people this kind of dangerous coagulating product, some of them are going to have [blood clots]."

Even though Holcomb, as the *New York Times* wrote, "understood the concerns of the Army's critics and agreed there was no strong evidence that the drug decreases mortality or other complications in trauma patients," he argued that the use of Factor Seven was justified because of the unique severity of the wounds in Iraq and Afghanistan. Among these were injuries caused by improvised explosive devices and roadside bombs, which meted out damage at a scale unlike anything seen in civilian hospitals. Soldiers in Humvees and trucks hit by bombs and explosive devices were, for example, getting both ripped open by shrapnel *and* burned after the vehicle ignited. The army argued that the devastation of these injuries required desperate measures—specifically the injection of Factor Seven into the arms of soldiers.

This argument was rejected by some doctors. "To say that because you're in a war, everything you do is right, suggests to me a level of arrogance that can only lead to a poor outcome," said Dr. Andrew Shorr, a former military critical care specialist. "Think about it," Shorr continued. "If you've got young soldiers having weirdo strokes, and you know they've been exposed to a drug like [Factor Seven], how long can you presume you don't have a safety issue? Just because you have the best of motives doesn't mean you don't have mediocre methods that are doing more harm than good. I don't believe that they don't have the capability to answer these questions. If you can't come to a conclusion, how do you come to the conclusion that it's safe?"

Here too Holcomb had a rejoinder. "You can't conduct clinical research in the middle of a war," he said in 2006. "We've been tracking patient outcomes as best we can. But we're in a setting where patients are moving across continents in the span of days. The data moves quickly. . . . It's not an excuse, it's just a fact." When it came to Factor Seven, Holcomb said, "We're not waiting" for more clinical research. "We'd still be talking about these things ten years from now."

But meanwhile, data that did not support the use of Factor Seven outside of hemophilia was piling up from highly credible sources. In February 2005 the *New England Journal of Medicine* published the results of the largest randomized clinical trial ever done on the drug. The study, conducted by Columbia University and funded by Novo Nordisk, involved four hundred patients, each of whom had suffered a hemorrhage in the brain. While Factor Seven significantly reduced bleeding, it was also significantly correlated with higher risk. Serious adverse events occurred in 2 percent of the placebo-treated patients, compared to 7 percent of the Factor Seven–treated patients. In October 2005 the FDA issued a warning against off-label use of the drug because of the risk of strokes and heart attacks. The warning was included in the package insert for the product. In January 2006, five months before Caleb Lufkin was injected with Factor Seven in Baghdad, FDA scientists published a review in *JAMA* that showed a long history of Factor Seven leading to strokes and heart attacks when used on people without hemophilia. The researchers reviewed adverse events after administration of Factor Seven that were reported to the FDA between 1999 and 2004, and they found that 185 blood clots and fifty deaths had occurred after off-label injections of the drug. The authors noted this figure was probably a gross underestimate, as reporting of adverse events was voluntary and historically captured only a fraction of the actual number of dangerous outcomes. Finally, in September 2006, the renowned R. Adams Cowley Shock Trauma Center in Baltimore published an analysis of patients given Factor Seven. It found an 8.7 percent rate of clot-related complications, which included twelve deaths partially attributed to the drug.

As these studies and reports were being published, the Israeli military, the original champion of using Factor Seven on soldiers, began pulling away from the drug. Michael Given went to a joint meeting in Tel Aviv with American and Israeli military surgeons and trauma specialists in 2006. At the meeting Israeli officials announced they were curtailing their use of the drug. Holcomb was at the meeting too. Given said later, "I recall John saying something like, 'But you're the guys who came up with this' and an Israeli doctor saying something like, 'I know, I know, but the data doesn't support it.'" The British military, which had used Factor Seven only minimally in the war, also stopped using the drug for anything but life-threatening bleeding which continued after all standard techniques had been exhausted. In an article announcing the policy change, doctors from Britain's Royal Centre for Defence Medicine cited the Cowley study. They noted that one-third of the complications that patients had experienced were associated with the drug itself, a percentage the British doctors found "highly consistent" with other large Factor Seven trials.

But Holcomb and the US Army chose to move forward with Factor Seven despite the accumulating data. In June 2005, Holcomb wrote in the *Journal of Trauma*, "In the 14 years Factor Seven has been clinically used, only a few cases of myocardial infarction [heart attack] and stroke have occurred." Remarkably, he told the *New York Times* in 2006, "You have a drug you know is safe from the prospective randomized controlled clinical trials. And you have to make a decision. It's not something you can decide to talk about. It's really yes or no. You have a lot of people bleeding to death in Iraq." Driven and as filled with certainty as always, Holcomb remained entirely committed to his vision, no matter what the FDA, the *New England Journal of Medicine*, and *JAMA* were saying. In making such pronouncements, Holcomb was staying entirely true to the definition of the ideal combat surgeon he had given at the RAND conference in Santa Monica back in 2000: a doctor with "good hands, a stout heart, and not too much philosophy" who is "called upon for decisions rather than discussion, for action rather than knowledge of what the latest writers think should be done."

The early adoption of Factor Seven by the army conferred upon the drug a kind of incalculable credibility. The military is one of America's most trusted institutions, especially in times of war. Despite the fact that there was still no FDA approval for Factor Seven beyond hemophilia, civilian trauma hospitals and centers around the country took notice of the army's adoption of the drug and began to introduce Factor Seven into their own facilities for general trauma victims.

Unsurprisingly, the army's embrace of Factor Seven coincided with an astounding rise in the drug's sales: between 2000 and 2008, for hospitalized patients without hemophilia, prescriptions for Factor Seven increased more than 140 times. By 2008, people with hemophilia accounted for only 3 percent of the drug's in-hospital use, while an extraordinary 97 percent of its use was for off-label indications.

By 2008, Factor Seven, which had had such a humble and obscure origin—young Ulla Hedner trying to treat six hemophilia patients with inhibitors in Sweden—became that elusive thing, a blockbuster drug with $1 billion a year in sales. John Holcomb and the United States Army had helped turn an orphan drug into a blockbuster, and it had helped Novo Nordisk make billions of dollars from the once obscure business of blood clotting.

––––––

When Private Caleb Lufkin was injected with Factor Seven on May 4, 2006, he of course had no idea about the long and controversial history of the drug. In fact, his family would not even learn that he had been given the drug until after his death, and they would hear of it only secondhand, through a media report, not from the army itself.

As Lufkin was being treated by the team in the Tenth Combat Support Hospital, the scene was observed by Robert Little, the war reporter and national correspondent for the *Baltimore Sun*. Little was a local Baltimore boy who had made good. At age thirteen he had delivered the newspaper on his bicycle. For the past few years he had been covering national defense issues for the *Sun*, and he had gotten to know John Holcomb quite well through his stories on national defense issues. Little had published an article in March 2005 in which he had reported favorably on Holcomb's advocacy for tourniquets in the war zone. Tens of thousands of army soldiers had been sent to war without them, and starting in 2002, Holcomb had pushed aggressively for the use of a new, lightweight tourniquet. Little's piece caused a furor on Capitol Hill, and the army responded by sending an additional 172,000 new-generation tourniquets to its soldiers.

Robert Little observed the course of Caleb Lufkin's surgery and treatment, as well as other events that transpired over the next few days in the Tenth Combat Support Hospital, and would later report on them in the *Baltimore Sun*. Lufkin's surgery seemed to go well enough, and the next day he was put on a helicopter and flown to Landstuhl in Germany. At almost exactly the time Lufkin was leaving, a wounded army captain named Shane Mahaffee arrived at the combat hospital and was brought to the emergency room.

Mahaffee was a thirty-six-year-old attorney with a small general law practice in Gurnee, Illinois, and was married with two young children. He was known for his wicked sense of humor, his exuberant personality, and his ability to light up a room at social events. Mahaffee, who had thick dark hair and a rugged athletic build, had served in the army reserves as a young man and retired in 1999, but he was eligible for reactivation. In October 2005 a FedEx package from the Department of Defense arrived at his home, summoning him to Iraq.

Like Lufkin, Mahaffee had been in a vehicle, in this case a Humvee, that was blown up by a bomb. Mahaffee, along with four other soldiers, had been in the lead Humvee in a convoy on a rural road sixty miles south of Baghdad. One of the soldiers, the gunner, saw what he believed might be a roadside bomb ahead of them. Should they stop or try to drive past it? No one in the vehicle quite seemed to know. Mahaffee called over the radio system to a commanding officer for advice, but just as he did, the driver, either confused or distracted, continued to move the Humvee forward. The other soldiers yelled at him to stop. But at this point they seemed so close that Mahaffee, the senior officer among them, cried, "Floor it!"

Two soldiers were killed instantly, and the driver was mortally wounded. Right after the bomb went off, the driver cried out, "I'm sorry! I'm sorry!" Mahaffee managed to escape the vehicle and attempted to walk and defend himself against the enemy. A soldier later said, "He was talking about setting up a security perimeter when one of the enlisted men had to tell him to lie down so he could treat him."

Mahaffee too was airlifted to the Tenth Combat Support Hospital. His hand was a pulp, and like Lufkin the day before, he was given plasma and blood, sedated, and put on a breathing tube. At first doctors didn't see any obvious bleeding, but X-rays revealed that he was hemorrhaging internally. Doctors gave him Factor Seven. "He needs it," one of the attending physicians said, "because he's going to bleed like hell." Blood filled his breathing tube. Doctors believed the bleeding was coming from Mahaffee's lung, so they made a huge incision in his chest, grasped the left lung, and twisted it, hoping this would halt the bleeding. By this point he had lost half of his blood. During the subsequent surgery, Mahaffee was given two more doses of Factor Seven, despite tests showing his clotting capacity was normal. His anesthesiologist justified the decision this way: "With these poly-trauma patients, once they start to get oozy, they can just spiral downhill. You can't wait for that to happen."

Mahaffee was awake only a few hours after surgery. In gratitude, he wrote a thank-you note on a clipboard for the hospital staff. To a fellow soldier in his unit, he scrawled, "Tell the guys I'm OK." To others in his unit, he wrote, "This job is not done." In yet another note he joked, "Hold all calls."

Like Lufkin before him, Mahaffee was flown to Germany. There he seemed to stabilize, and he was scheduled to fly back to the United States. But the day before he was supposed to leave, a blood clot appeared in his lung. He became unconscious and was put on a ventilator. He died on May 15, eight days after the bombing.

Mahaffee's death was attributed to complications of pneumonia and infection, but as Robert Little later wrote in the *Baltimore Sun*, "His doctors said it was the ventilator that likely prompted the infection, and it was the clot that put him on the ventilator." Doctors said he probably would have survived his injuries in Iraq if he hadn't suffered the blood clot. "I had a very bad feeling about his injury from the beginning," said Mahaffee's widow. "I don't know why. Even when other people were being optimistic, I just didn't think he was ever going to come back."

His father, Skip Mahaffee, said that five thousand people attended his son's funeral in Illinois on May 22, 2006. "We paid dearly for our freedom, and it's not paid with gold or money. It's paid with American blood," Skip Mahaffee would later say.

Caleb Lufkin too would soon have a funeral in Illinois. The day after Lufkin arrived at Landstuhl, he was flown to Walter Reed in

Bethesda. His mother, a nurse in a cardiac unit, came to visit him at Walter Reed on May 8—having taken the first airplane flight of her life—and was horrified at what she witnessed upon arrival. Her son's injuries were more severe than she'd expected, and she was disturbed by the glassy look in his eyes. She fed him with a spoon and cleaned the dirt from under his fingernails.

"Try to imagine walking through that door and seeing your perfect child lying there, blown apart, with cuts and pieces of shrapnel all over him and his eyes just lifeless," said Marcy Gorsline. "I'd never felt so angry before."

The sink in Lufkin's room kept clogging. At one point there was urine on the floor, and it would be hours before the staff came to address it. She cleaned it up herself. She said later, "After what these kids did for us, we can't even give them a clean room to recover in?"

On May 18 he underwent surgery to repair his left leg. But strangely, a blood clot appeared in Lufkin's lung during the procedure, and the operation was aborted. Lufkin had to be put on a respirator and transferred to intensive care. The doctors were mystified as to how a young person like Lufkin could develop such a clot. They decided to give him time to recover and scheduled a second surgery for a week later.

In the days before the second surgery, Caleb Lufkin was nervous but appeared reasonably assured. Doctors made discharge plans for him to go home to Illinois, where the plan was for him to commence physical therapy. From his bed he spoke of future plans, like a trip to Australia. He planned a cookout right down to the menu. His teenage brothers came to visit him, along with his grandmother and other family members, who fed him cookies and Subway sandwiches. Lufkin was in pain much of the time, and he suffered bouts of intolerable itching, but he seemed to be gradually doing better. "He was starting to finally come to life," Gorsline said. "He could see an end to all of it."

The second surgery was scheduled for May 25, and all was expected to go well. Caleb's mother was doing a crossword puzzle in the lobby when a team of doctors and counselors invited her into a private room, then told her that her son had gone into cardiac arrest on the operating table and died. "No one's ever been able to explain to me how someone so young and so healthy could die of a heart attack like that." His army autopsy reported only that Lufkin had perished of complications of injuries from a bomb blast.

Tammy Lufkin, Caleb's father, heard that his son had been injected with Factor Seven only when one of his customers at the lumberyard in Illinois told him. The patron had read news reports, presumably written by Robert Little, about the use of the drug on Caleb. Tammy Lufkin said, "I am so upset that I didn't know that they'd given him Factor Seven....When he was at Walter Reed and his arms were always swelling up and he was itching like crazy, I was asking them a million questions and they didn't tell me anything." He added, "I can't bring my kid back but maybe we can get somebody to take responsibility."

Tammy Lufkin approached lawyers to discuss whether, because it had used Factor Seven, the Department of Defense was responsible for his son's death. "I don't care if we get a dime out of it," he said. "I don't know lawyer stuff. I just want someone to take responsibility. You can't keep pushing the buck on somebody else." But any good lawyer would have told Mr. Lufkin that his pursuit was fruitless because of the Feres doctrine, which prevents soldiers from suing the US government over battlefield injuries.

At Caleb Lufkin's funeral in Galesburg, Illinois, on June 2, members of the Westboro Baptist Church disrupted the proceedings. Members of this group believe that the United States is being punished for sins such as homosexuality and adultery and that dead soldiers are evidence of God's wrath. A group of protesters from Westboro held signs, and children and teens sang, "Filthy fags, God hates you."

Caleb's mother had chosen a grave site near a flagpole. "I looked up and saw that flag flying and said, 'I want him right here, right under that flag,'" Gorsline said. "He died for that flag, and everyone who comes here will hear it flapping in the wind." A tree was also planted at Lufkin's high school in his honor. But in 2014 the tree was unintentionally cut down during construction at the school. Two years later, a new oak tree was planted, and an engraved granite memorial dedicated to Lufkin was installed across from the baseball field where he had played left field and worn number 15.

In December 2006 the *Baltimore Sun* ran Little's article on Mahaffee's and Lufkin's deaths. It included deep reporting on Factor Seven and its risks, and it was one article in a series that also included stories on the controversy around HemCon and QuikClot. These would represent the first comprehensive national reporting on the race between the agents for stemming volume bleeding on the battlefield. But it was the piece on Lufkin's and Mahaffee's deaths, entitled "Don't Let Me Die," that attracted by far the most attention. The article led to immediate calls for an investigation into the army's, and in particular John Holcomb's, use of Factor Seven.

Only two weeks after the article was published, John Holcomb was asked to appear before a Senate subcommittee to explain why exactly the army had adopted Factor Seven in the first place.

CHAPTER NINE

Emotional Bankruptcy

IN DECEMBER 2006, in his home in the "Pfizer ghetto" in Niantic, Bart Gullong read the stories of Caleb Lufkin's and Shane Mahaffee's deaths in the *Baltimore Sun* while sitting at the breakfast table and was filled with apoplectic rage. He could hardly bring himself to speak when Linda asked him what was wrong. Bart previously had absolutely no idea of the extent of the army's use of Factor Seven. Nor had he been aware of the expense and risks associated with the drug. That the army had declined to adopt QuikClot despite its documented success and had instead thrown in its lot with an untested drug that cost up to $10,000 a dose and might be killing soldiers was simply inconceivable to Bart. It made him even more outraged than he already was that he had been attacked so much for QuikClot. The absolute worst things that QuikClot could cause were relatively short-lived, if intense, pain and a significant burn that would heal in a couple of weeks—not a fatal heart attack or stroke. Frank was appalled by the *Baltimore Sun* articles too, but, as always, didn't carry the burden the way Bart did; Frank, after all, was a sanguine soul, and most of the time he was able to shrug things off with a laugh and go back to tinkering with gas pressures. But Bart couldn't let it go. His outrage grew even deeper when a defense industry publication reported that QuikClot had saved 150 lives in Iraq and Afghanistan by 2006. His reaction was fueled even further when he considered that for some time now—in the scuttlebutt that surrounded the medical conferences—he and Frank had been called "war profiteers," ambulance chasers making a filthy buck off the lives of soldiers and the American military machine.

After the articles were published, Bart—who had never been the easiest person to work or live with in the first place—became steadily edgier. At work he began to snap at his employees, swearing at the workers on the factory floor at the slightest mistake and screaming at the secretaries. Tensions with Steven, the CEO, with whom he'd always had a fraught relationship, grew intolerable. Most days Bart would go into his office, shut the door behind him, and isolate for hours. His once-formidable productivity plummeted, and there were entire mornings and afternoons when he just stared at his computer screen. At times Bart threw things around the office behind his closed door—papers, staplers, coffee cups. The staff heard the sounds of destruction from outside and learned not to intrude lest they get their heads handed to them. Bart virtually stopped attending the endless product trade shows that had dominated his life for the past few years. At the last one he attended, in Indianapolis, he had gotten so crazily depressed and drunk in his hotel room that he threw a liquor bottle out of a window. He was on the seventh floor, and it could have killed someone. In the morning he went to the courtyard and cleaned up the smashed detritus of the bottle—and was deeply ashamed.

At home his marriage was beginning to crumble. Linda resented his volatile moods and the increasing distance between them. She removed herself as much as she could from Bart, exploring her own interests, which were increasingly various New Age healing practices. They had less and less to say to each other, their sole remaining shared interest being their daughter, now ten, whom they both adored. Around Sarah's care, at least, Bart and Linda worked well together, collaborating on playdates, parent-teacher conferences, and homework help. Linda didn't really understand what had happened to Bart—and when she asked him what was going on, he wouldn't answer. He would just go into the den and watch sports and drink a Scotch. There were no big fights between them, simply a protracted cold war. Linda couldn't quite believe that just a few years before, Bart had been so full of life, so much fun—at the center of parties with their neighbors, building the massive float for the holiday parade on Main Street, and taking the family out almost every summer weekend to cruise the Long Island Sound in motorboats and sailboats and yachts.

In the last few years, Bart had been crushed under the weight of helping to run two companies, On-Site Gas *and* Z-Medica. As both grew and became more successful, there was of course more and more work. Frank was always the nine-to-five guy— at the end of each day, he would quietly drive home to West Hartford and Nancy and the kids. Steven at Z-Medica minded the shop but also had a very well-regulated and finite sense of his job. It was left to Bart to do all the travel and the big sales calls and meetings for both companies. It was therefore Bart whose cell phone was on 24/7 and who got calls from all over the world for orders in the middle of the night. And it was Bart who had worked almost alone with the navy and marines and mastered the intricacies of the military and who bore the brunt of the army's assault. Frank was involved, to be sure, but he almost always kept himself at a remove, and he was blessed with his usual equanimity, his Dale Carnegie power of positive thinking, and his enduring belief that everything would work out in the end. Bart did not think that everything was going to work out.

There was one particular task during this time—sometime in late 2006 or early 2007, although the weeks and months were beginning to merge into one another—that seemed to break Bart. The manual for the POGS machines needed revising. On the face of it, it was a simple enough job, a small project that a few years earlier he would have cranked out in a day or two. But Bart resented that he was the only one in the company who seemed capable of doing this. He would have liked to think that at this point in On-Site Gas's evolution, someone else could have handled it; after all, at this point the company had actual credentialed engineers on staff. But Bart found that if they understood the engineering, they couldn't write, and if they could write, they didn't fully understand the engineering. Bart, as usual, was the one to pick up the pieces. He worked in his closed office for days on the manual, seething. It took him one agonizing week to finish it.

Bart also realized that he was furious at Frank too. Somewhere along the line, a few years earlier, Frank had said that he would give Bart a 25 percent ownership share of On-Site. This seemed a deserved reward to Bart—after all, when he'd first arrived, the company had had a website featuring stick figures and a staff of three. But lately Frank had begun saying he would instead give Bart a one-time payout of $600,000 for his contributions. Certainly that was a lot of money, but it was in no way equivalent to one-quarter of a successful company with a promising future. That would be worth millions, eventually even tens of millions. Bart was pretty sure that Frank had not simply forgotten about this promise. He began to believe that Frank had backed off because he had lost faith in Bart, given his partner's newly strange and erratic behavior. That was crushing to Bart; they had accomplished so much together and worked so compatibly. And what hurt even more was that Bart knew that Frank's doubts about him were in some ways justified. He wanted to raise these issues with Frank, but he knew there was no point. Frank had a long history with business partners who had burned him. If Bart confronted him, he knew that Frank would not react well.

Throughout 2007, Bart felt himself beginning to crack. He started taking the antidepressant Lexapro, which helped some, but not much. Linda had begun saying that she wanted to move to Florida. She too was depressed, at least in the winter, from seasonal affective disorder, and she said she needed to get out of New England. Bart had always wanted to retire to Florida, but this move would be ten years ahead of schedule. But in an attempt to help Linda, and perhaps to save his marriage, he agreed to the purchase of a house in the gated community of Palm Beach Gardens, ten miles west of Palm Beach. Linda began going to the house for long weekends, bringing Sarah with her. But Bart felt obliged to stay in Connecticut and attempt to regain his standing with Frank and Z-Medica. The temporary separations from his family depressed Bart further.

But the real reason for the rapid decline in Bart's mental state was something that he could not share with anyone. When Bart was working on QuikClot and the POGS, senior government officials had been impressed with his entrepreneurial and administrative savvy. They'd asked him to lead a team on a contract basis to go "down range" in Iraq as a classified government contractor. There Bart led a team of specialists. What he did in Iraq was and remains protected information, but it amounted to assisting with defensive—not offensive—strategy, and to function in a completely nonmilitary role. Bart was stunned that he had been asked to take on this role and gratified by the opportunity to serve his country. He was offered payment but refused it. He considered the job to be his patriotic duty, and he had always considered himself patriotic, even—or perhaps especially—when he was protesting the Vietnam War. This recognition of his expertise at the very highest levels of government was enough. On the ground in Iraq, he was deeply moved at the presence of QuikClot in the field, which was available to both Americans and Iraqis, including civilians. After all, there were far more Iraqis being killed and wounded in the war than Americans—later estimates were that the number of Iraqi deaths, astoundingly, had been about thirty times greater than those suffered by the US military.

The terms of his consulting contract were such that it was extremely confidential, and he could not tell Frank about it, or even Linda. He would get a call from the higher-ups, usually with virtually no notice, telling him that he needed to go to Iraq. He would simply say to Linda that he had to go somewhere for a few days and would be back. At this point in their dissolving marriage, Linda thought he was having an affair, and she would merely nod. To Frank, Bart would say that he had some pressing personal business and wouldn't be coming into the office for a little bit. And then Bart would be flown to Iraq via a combination of commercial and military air transport.

When in Iraq, he would ride in a vehicle across the desert. Bart was almost always jet-lagged, disoriented, and uncomfortable, but at the same time he believed there was something beautiful about the journey he was undertaking: the surprisingly straight tarmac road sailing across the near empty desert, the vast expanse interrupted only by the occasional palm tree or boxy concrete house or store.

He felt almost happy to be there, away from the turmoil at home. There was something gorgeous about the desert and its soaring, endless turquoise sky. It reminded him of sailing the deep Atlantic waters off Montauk when he'd lived on the east end of Long Island. But he also saw casualties of war and bodies torn apart by bombs, arms and limbs separated from torsos lying on the ground. It was ghastly beyond anything he had ever witnessed, or even imagined. Firsthand, Bart experienced the terror of life "outside the wire." In Iraq, one could be sitting one moment at a café and then killed the next moment by flying glass after a bomb blast. He experienced the death-at-any-moment reality that soldiers and civilians alike faced. It shook Bart deeply, but unlike the combatants he was there only for very short periods. After a few days, his assignment would be up. He returned to work at Z-Medica, unable to reveal anything he had seen. In the way of the upper reaches of the government, he was never told the number of casualties that might have occurred in the carnage he witnessed.

One day not long after Bart had experienced such an episode and was back home, Frank came into the office and saw Bart staring at the holly bushes outside the window and quietly crying. It was just so strange to Frank that the man who had been so ebullient and voluble—who could talk to anyone, and usually talk circles around them—and who had relentlessly traveled around the country three or four days a week, transforming his company, could now be this shell in front of him. This was the same man who had worked sometimes sixteen hours straight, increasing their salaries to almost $1 million each within three years of his arrival in 1999. Now everyone in the building—twenty employees, many of whom Frank considered friends more than employees—wanted Bart to leave, at least for a while, even if they were too afraid to say it.

Frank knew that Bart must be having some kind of breakdown,

but it was not Frank's style to ask him directly about it. Frank's response to Bart's erratic behavior was mainly to avoid him. But they did still meet one day a week to go over progress and orders and strategy, and to review the "booked-to-build" log as they had in the old days. Frank would make vague mentions of concern or ask Bart two or three times during a meeting, "How are you doing?" in a pointed way that was unusual for him. In response, Bart would say, "I'm fine, Frank. Just fine."

Sometime in 2007, Frank called Bart into his office. As they spoke, Frank was mainly looking down, avoiding eye contact. He told Bart that it might be a good idea if Bart took a little break.

"Why don't you go to Florida for a bit," Frank said brightly. "Take a break! You've earned it." Then Frank said, again, "Just be a consultant for a while. We'll have to reduce your pay—not much—but you should take a break for a while. Be with your family."

The way Frank said it, Bart knew it was an order, or as close to an order as Frank could muster. As much as they were partners, Frank was still ultimately his boss. And Frank had made it clear he wanted Bart to leave. Frank had always liked Linda, the way he liked just about everyone he knew, and he believed that it would be best for Linda and Bart to be together. Whatever was ailing Bart, it was probably nothing that spending some time away in the sun with his wife couldn't fix.

Bart walked, stunned, out of the meeting—which had taken all of five minutes. He shouldn't have cared at this point, but even amid the shock of the news and his own tumultuous mental state, he worried about what was going to happen to Z-Medica. But Bart also realized that Frank was ultimately right to ask him to leave. It was a matter of his survival. And it helped too that Linda was delighted about this development. She saw it as a way to save her marriage and her family—they could all be together happily in

Florida, where it would be 70 degrees in February. And as much as he seethed at what amounted in some ways to a kind of firing, one piece of Bart agreed with the decision, at least on a strategic basis. Bart had always been the face of QuikClot to the military, and therefore the chief antagonist against Holcomb. To the army Bart was the enemy. His disappearance for a while might help the product. If stepping away helped QuikClot, and helped save more lives, then Bart was willing to do so, at least for some period of time. He had always said that the product should run the company, not the other way around. But with a terrible sinking feeling, he also realized that he had regressed to his mean, reliving the historical pattern that had defined his life—undertaking brilliant work for three or four years and then slinking away to the next thing.

In late 2007 the family moved full-time to Florida. There he tried to take on the new semitropical lifestyle—sailing, fishing, and golf—but nothing seemed to take. He and Linda went to counseling but Bart continued to be difficult at home. His mood did not improve, and Linda seemed to avoid him just as much as she had in Connecticut, going to the beach, hanging out with friends, anything to get out of the house. Purportedly Bart worked on strategy for Z-Medica from afar, but most of his days were just as murky as they had been in Connecticut. After a few months, things were so bad with Linda that she would often leave the house to stay with a girlfriend a town away.

One afternoon when Bart lay on the couch, it all came rushing back to him at once: the bombs in Iraq, the sounds of blasts that defied the limitations of reality, the dawning awareness that he and a lot of other people could have died in the desert. While in the field he had been calm, but now he began to shake. It was a year-long delayed reaction. Images continued to flood his brain, all accompanied by fear and depression. And once it had been unleashed, it wouldn't go away. It went on and on, in the afternoons and in the dark nights ahead. But over the weeks, the images began to change; the violence of Iraq became charged with the violence of his father, and then the withering arrogance of John Holcomb on that phone call in which he had laughed at Bart, the sounds and images bleeding into each other.

At the house in Palm Beach Gardens, he would sit for seven hours on the couch and watch television. *Deadliest Catch* was an old standby, but it didn't really matter what was on. He just needed something to distract him from the thoughts in his head. He would have soda and potato chips for lunch and stale pizza for dinner.

He never thought about killing himself—he knew, thankfully, that he was too narcissistic to do that.

It was a mystery to everyone, even to Bart, why exactly he was so broken. He thought back on his vitality, the days when he had been a rower and a coach who built championship teams. Had he told his fifty-five-year-old self ten years before that he would turn On-Site Gas around, create a new company, and bring to market a product that would save lives, he would have been flabbergasted. He had fulfilled the promise he'd made to himself around the time that he first met Frank at Paradise Pizza—that he was going to no longer be Willy Loman, a salesman with nothing to sell. He had truly reached his potential for the first time in his life, and he had learned what he was destined to be—a socially conscious entrepreneur. He should have been proud. But it didn't matter how much he had achieved or how much money he had in the bank: he had become emotionally bankrupt.

The images and voices came to him with no warning, in the middle of the night, or the moment *Deadliest Catch* went off the air. First it would be his father's face, and his father's voice: aggressive, lacerating, torturing: *You thought you were a man, but you're just a foolish little boy*. Over and over again, the voices forming an echo chamber of disgust. Whatever Bart had achieved in his teens, twenties, thirties was all just fodder for his father's ongoing evisceration. The irony was that his father, on the face of it, was an admirable enough character. The neighbors who had attended his barbecues at Cornfield Point might have thought he was OK. He dutifully waved hello to them while mowing his lawn, or while he hoisted all the right patriotic and maritime flags in the yard on all the right holidays. He had served his country in World War II, taken care materially of his family, dutifully punched the clock at the engineering company for thirty years, paid the tuition bills. But at the end of it all, he was a hateful man. The neighbors didn't know about Bart's father's depression, or his acid nature, and how he seemed to gain strength from tearing his son down. He had never once told Bart he was proud of him, or loved him, or even liked him. There had been only one such moment, as his father lay dying in a hospital after a heart attack when Bart was in his late forties. His father had said, weakly, "You know, Barton"—his father always called him Barton—"I was pretty hard on you…" Bart knew in that moment that the decades of vituperation could be wiped out with a single honest sentence. Bart, like a child, hung on every word, waiting to hear what he believed would be some kind of apology. Whatever was to come had the potential to change the arc of their relationship, and even perhaps the balance of Bart's life. But Bart's sister swept in, rolling her eyes, cutting her father off. "Come on!" she said, leaving the wished-for apology forever unrealized. His father died hours later.

As he spent months on the couch in Florida in 2008, Bart came to believe he might be suffering from post-traumatic stress disorder from all he had endured, and indeed a clinician whom he saw briefly in Florida said he had delayed PTSD from what he had witnessed in Iraq. And that's what Bart thought too, at first. But that, he began to realize, was wrong. He was suffering from PTSD from a lifetime of hounding by his father followed by the destruction of his achievement by the army in its arrogance. These things had led to Bart being alone on a couch in a dark-shadowed living room in the brilliance of a sunlit Florida afternoon. It was just as he used to tell his young rowers when he was a coach. The art of winning involves taking on more pain than the other person. If you could take the most pain, you could win. But here Bart was taking more pain than anyone, but it was all for nothing.

No, Bart realized. The ultimate source of his pain wasn't what he'd experienced in Iraq. It wasn't his ire over Caleb Lufkin. It wasn't even really John Holcomb. No, the ultimate source of pain was himself.

PART THREE

THE FINISH LINE

Pain? Yes, of course. Racing without pain is
not racing. But the pleasure of being ahead
outweighed the pain a million times over. To
hell with the pain. What's six minutes of pain
compared to the pain they're going to feel for
the next six months or six decades?

—Brad Alan Lewis, United States gold
medalist in rowing, 1984 Olympic games

CHAPTER TEN

United States v. Novo Nordisk

A WEEK AFTER Robert Little's *Baltimore Sun* articles about Caleb Lufkin and Shane Mahaffee were published in December 2006, and while Bart was still in Niantic and a year away from moving to Florida, the Democratic senator from Maryland, Barbara Mikulski, wrote a letter to the assistant secretary of defense for health affairs. It read in part as follows:

> I urge you to immediately review the use and effects of this drug, known as Factor VII. As a member of the Defense Sub-committee of the Senate Appropriations Committee...the serious questions that have been raised about Factor VII must be answered....It is important to know whether Factor VII patients are more prone to blood clots or other complications, which may not develop in the first hours or days after initial treatment. We need to know if the long-term risks of this drug pose a greater danger to our service member's [sic] lives than can be justified by the short-term benefits.

Additionally, Senate Minority Whip Dick Durbin said that the articles had prompted him to seek similar answers from Pentagon officials. "The safety of our troops is the top priority and my office is discussing the serious findings reported in the *Baltimore Sun* with the Defense Department," the Illinois Democrat said.

There was no public response from the army to the Mikulski letter or Durbin's concerns. But John Holcomb was called to Capitol Hill to testify to the Defense Subcommittee. He presented a PowerPoint on December 7, 2006, only a few weeks after Little's articles were published. In a characteristic matter-of-fact manner, he stated right at the beginning of his presentation the main point that he wanted to make. He wrote:

BOTTOM LINE UP FRONT

rFVIIa is part of the data-driven, experience based, comprehensive, integrated improvements in trauma management during GWOT [Global War on Terrorism]

Complications occur in seriously injured patients. Based on our continuing analysis of clinical data, we believe the benefits of rFVIIa outweigh the potential risks.

He went on to indicate, "At no time have we seen increases in complications among those treated, compared to untreated, either in the literature or in our experience." He summarized by saying, "We are using the drug appropriately."

In his remarks Holcomb cited, among others, the 2005 study in the *New England Journal of Medicine* that found elevated adverse events associated with Factor Seven, but he neglected to mention the FDA's 2005 warning about Factor Seven for uses outside of hemophilia, or the FDA studies that had shown hundreds of serious complications from the drug. Holcomb maintained the position he'd taken at the RAND Corporation in 2000—that the FDA has no place on the battlefield.

There is no specific evidence anywhere that Holcomb's appearance before the committee directly led to a change in practice. In fact there is no available documentation of the committee's response to the presentation. Barbara Mikulski's papers are currently stored in the Sheridan Libraries at Johns Hopkins University, and while they contain records about Factor Seven, they are, according to the archivist, "closed for research until 2032." However, coincidentally or not, the use of Factor Seven in the war zone dramatically decreased after Holcomb's appearance on Capitol Hill, as it did in civilian practice for trauma. In 2006, Robert Little had witnessed a dozen doses of Factor Seven injected in a single day at the Tenth Combat Support Hospital, but at the same hospital in 2008, it was used a dozen times in six months. In 2007 the British military essentially stopped using Factor Seven. Dr. Alam, now at the influential Massachusetts General Hospital in Boston, said that "the hospital stopped using it almost entirely. The results of those clinical trials just killed the drug." These days, Factor Seven is almost completely out of favor in trauma medicine and hardly ever used. Its use in trauma is now a historic, and largely closed, episode.

In 2016, Demetrios Demetriades, the internationally famous hematologist, said as much in a lecture. Demetriades captured the entire Factor Seven story with the following pithy anecdote:

[Factor Seven] was born in 1999 from a case report. It was in Israel, there was a soldier with a gunshot injury, he was bleeding a lot. They couldn't stop the bleeding; they didn't despair; one of the surgeons gave Factor Seven. And for some reason, the bleeding stopped. The bleeding stopped because...nobody knows. But he attributed this to Factor Seven. On the basis of one case—poorly documented case—the whole practice changed! All the trauma centers were using Factor Seven left and right. You need two doses, and the price for that was $17,000. The military, at one stage, they ran out of Factor Seven. The military bought all the stocks because they were preparing for war. We couldn't find it. Unbelievable. Well guess what? In 2005, this concept died from a randomized study. They did a randomized study; it says it does not really help. Classic example of quickly adopted [sic] a scientifically unproven concept.

The fall of Factor Seven coincided with another downward spiral: that of John Holcomb's career as the leader of army trauma medicine. For some time there had been growing complaints about Holcomb's conduct at the Institute of Surgical Research. In a March 12, 2007, memo to the inspector general of the army, who oversees internal investigations, colleagues accused Holcomb of "initiating numerous and consistent actions of mismanagement and misuse of authority and funding associated within his function." The writers pointed out that Holcomb had recommended HemCon for use on the battlefield despite unpublished studies showing that it was not statistically significantly more effective than standard gauze, and that he'd then submitted HemCon, under his name, as one of the army's "Greatest Inventions of 2004." A later memo references colleagues' concerns that the Institute of Surgical Research under Holcomb "stressed results at the expense of good science." Another expressed a deep ambivalence about Holcomb: in a single sentence, an officer at the institute referred to him as both "arrogant, obnoxious, [and] overbearing" and "exactly the type of leader the ISR needed." The inspector general commenced a formal investigation into Holcomb's performance as commander of the institute but a report issued in December 2007 cleared Holcomb and the ISR of any wrongdoing.

Nonetheless, John Holcomb's end with the military came with surprising quickness. Citing the stress of the investigation, John Holcomb resigned as commander of the Institute of Surgical Research in the summer of 2008. A formal change of command ceremony was held at the Center for the Intrepid at Fort Sam Houston in San Antonio. Holcomb was awarded a medal reserved for those who have made outstanding contributions to special operations by Admiral Eric Olson, commander of US Special Operations Command. Another colonel, also a medical doctor, immediately took over leadership of the institute. It all transpired rather quietly. Bart and Frank did not even hear about Holcomb's separation from the military until several months after it happened.

But just as quickly, Holcomb landed on his feet. Almost immediately after his resignation, he became a professor of surgery at the University of Texas's Medical School in Austin, where he held multiple titles, all of them impressive sounding: director at the Center for Translational Injury Research, chief of acute care surgery, and vice chair of the department of surgery. Holcomb began his career at the University of Texas with the same passion and workaholic energy he had brought to the Institute of Surgical Research. He soon became the face of the hospital in high-profile cases and studies involving trauma medicine. He would say years later, with his characteristic combination of optimism and hubris, "We've been able to reduce the number of trauma deaths at our hospital by thirty percent just by applying the skills I learned in the military."

But there was more trouble lurking for Holcomb in 2008. Major Ian Black, an anesthesiologist who had worked under him in combat hospitals in Iraq and as a researcher at the Institute of Surgical Research, filed a complaint with the army's inspector general on the day he resigned from active duty in the army. He asked the inspector general to investigate the army's use of Factor Seven. Dr. Black filed the complaint on the day of his resignation because he feared retaliation from his former superiors.

Then, additionally, on October 31, 2008, Dr. Black filed a major whistleblower lawsuit against Novo Nordisk in the District Court of Maryland. The lawsuit was delivered to the Edward A. Garmatz United States District Courthouse, a seventies-era modernist office building made of glass and concrete, and it would lead to a three-year legal dispute in which John Holcomb and the Institute of Surgical Research were heavily implicated.

In 2008, Ian Black was a relatively young doctor. He had graduated from Pennsylvania State University College of Medicine in 1999, his tuition paid for by the army, and then completed his internship at Brooke Army Medical Center in San Antonio, which was closely affiliated with the Institute of Surgical Research. After finishing his internship in 2003, he rose through army medicine to become the lead anesthesiologist at the burn center at Brooke. In some ways Black appeared to be the classic military doctor—athletic in build, optimistic, and outspoken by nature. But there was another aspect to him, a Renaissance man quality, that was perhaps less typical. He spoke French, Spanish, and Arabic, published poetry, and wrote thoughtful personal reflections in medical journals. After the war started, he gave an in-depth interview to National Public Radio's *All Things Considered*. In the interview he described the burn center as "a cornucopia of pain" and talked about "the hubris" involved in even presuming to understand what his patients were going through. In the range of his interests, Black was rather similar to Joe Dacorta, with whom he became friendly. They often connected at the trauma medicine conferences over their shared grievances with the system.

Early on, Black had used Factor Seven occasionally on patients suffering from massive bleeding. His suspicions were aroused October 2005 when he was put up at the Ritz-Carlton in Atlanta and given lavish dinners, all paid for by Novo Nordisk, to attend a medical meeting. Black was surprised that Novo Nordisk treated him as if he were an authority on Factor Seven; in reality he was a young doctor with limited experience. Many years later, reflecting on the experience, Black said, "They asked me if I used the drug. I said yes. They said, 'Good, you're an expert.'" He began to suspect that he was being manipulated by the drug company. "And I guess I had a little bit of an epiphany that oh my God, these guys are playing me," he said.

In December 2006 Black was in Iraq, working at the Twenty-Eighth Combat Support Hospital in Baghdad. This was one of the peaks of the war, and he "was tired beyond words." Black was then treating hundreds of maimed and dying soldiers and civilians—men, women, and children. The injuries were horrific: multiple missing limbs, bodies riddled with bullets. In a matter of weeks he treated a man who had been set on fire, a contractor who had had both arms blown off, and an Iraqi official's wife whose eyes had been shot out during an assassination attempt on her husband. A mortuary officer he worked with had stopped eating because she was overwhelmed from stacking dead bodies. The clogs he wore in the operating room had become rotten from the amount of time he'd spent standing in blood. Eventually he had to wear galoshes. In 2008 Black wrote, "I won't miss keeping the mortally wounded alive long enough so their spouse, or child, or parents can try to take their leave a little closer to home. . . . I will miss working with patients who comfort their mother on the telephone from a hospital bed: 'Don't worry, Mama, it was only a leg. I'll be all right.'"

In Iraq in 2006, he was stunned by how liberally Factor Seven was being dispensed in combat hospitals, including to those not bleeding badly, and he witnessed two patients suffer from embolisms after being given the drug. He also saw a distressing lack of checks and balances in the system that governed army trauma medicine. As commander of the institute, Holcomb was largely unilaterally in charge of both research and clinical practice guidelines. Black was also troubled by the lack of serious studies into Factor Seven's impact on trauma patients. He was alarmed by the FDA's study on Factor Seven, which reported 185 thromboembolic events, such as strokes and heart attacks, linked to the drug. Black said, "It didn't mean for sure it caused it, but it certainly gave me pause."

While in Iraq, Black was ordered to do a study of clinical practice guidelines and make recommendations, and he proposed greatly curtailing Factor Seven's use. Black and his fellow doctors transmitted their proposal up the medical chain of command, but their suggestions were never formally adopted, and they didn't appear to get much of a response. Nonetheless, Black and other doctors dramatically cut back on their use of Factor Seven. And they observed that the survival rate of patients in their hospital remained the same even after this dramatic reduction.

Black, however, did receive an angry phone call from John Holcomb, who was incensed about not seeing Black's proposal before it was shared with others. Given the tone of the conversation and their differing opinions on Factor Seven, Black suggested to Holcomb that he (Black) not return to work at the Institute of Surgical Research. To that Holcomb agreed.

It was subsequent to that dispute that Black filed the complaint to the army inspector general and then the federal whistleblower lawsuit in Baltimore. At the crux of the lawsuit were two central allegations: that he and other doctors had felt pressured to use Factor Seven by Novo Nordisk, and that kickbacks from the drug company to physicians had occurred.

Ian Black was joined in the whistleblower lawsuit by Dr. Oscar Montiel, who had worked for Novo Nordisk in its West Texas and Oklahoma regions as a medical science liaison from October 2004 to May 2006. Medical science liaisons play a vital role within a pharmaceutical company. The position often requires a doctorate in the life sciences, and such liaisons often act as a critical bridge between a drug company and prescribing physicians. Often the main role of the medical science liaison is building relationships with "key opinion leaders," or physicians prominent in their fields. Montiel alleged that Novo Nordisk had conducted illegal marketing schemes to promote Factor Seven to army physicians.

Black was represented by Dan Hargrove, a San Antonio attorney with a small practice. Hargrove, a former air force reserve judge advocate—military judge advocates provide legal counsel within their respective military branch—had held the rank of lieutenant colonel and had taught law at the US Army's Judge Advocate General's Legal Center and School at the University of Virginia. Montiel was represented by a much larger national firm, Waters Kraus & Paul, which had an office in Baltimore. This firm mainly focused on work-related illnesses and injuries, dangerous drugs, and exposure to harmful chemicals and other toxic substances, but it also had experience with whistleblower lawsuits.

Montiel and Black sued Novo Nordisk under the provisions of the False Claims Act, a federal law that imposes liability on people and entities who defraud the federal government. The False Claims Act is often called the Lincoln Law because it was passed during Abraham Lincoln's presidency to combat fraud during the Civil War, which was rampant throughout both the Union and the Confederacy. For example, contractors sold sick horses and mules, malfunctioning rifles, and spoiled provisions to the Union Army. The most significant case involving the False Claims Act—which Black, Montiel, Hargrove, and Waters Kraus & Paul were surely well aware of—was brought against the drug company Parke-Davis in 1996. At one time Parke-Davis was the largest pharmaceutical company in the world, sometimes called "the pride of Detroit." The 1996 case concerned the company's off-label marketing scheme for Neurontin, a drug approved for epilepsy treatment but used off-label for pain management as well as to treat bipolar disorder and attention deficit hyperactivity disorder. Just like Oscar Montiel, David Franklin, the whistleblower, worked as a medical liaison for Parke-Davis. He alleged that doctors were paid kickbacks for prescribing large amounts of Neurontin and given gifts such as travel and tickets to the Olympics. Parke-Davis also paid doctors to release confidential information about their patients who had received Neurontin. The company destroyed evidence and falsified papers in order to conceal its off-label marketing scheme from the FDA. Parke-Davis paid $430 million in fines to the government, and Franklin himself received $24 million.

Ian Black and Oscar Montiel were joined by the United States Department of Justice and twenty-three states in their complaint against Novo Nordisk. The fact that the Department of Justice had chosen to lead the case spoke to the credibility of Black's and Montiel's allegations; the federal government, generally picking the ones it believes it can win, declines to represent the vast majority of False Claims Act cases. Still, a great deal was riding on the outcome of the case for Ian Black and Oscar Montiel beyond their professional credibility and fear of reprisals. Under the terms of the False Claims Act, whistleblowers receive between 15 and 30 percent of any awards. But it would take a full three years before they would learn the outcome.

The lawsuit claimed, as CBS News later reported, that Novo Nordisk illegally funded medical experiments on injured soldiers in Iraq in order to widen the use of Factor Seven. In fact, experimenting on soldiers injured in battle is illegal. Only the US president is able to sign a waiver that allows research drugs to be used on American soldiers during a time of war. The suit specifically alleged that Novo Nordisk promoted Factor Seven to US Army doctors and researchers at the Institute of Surgical Research, which included John Holcomb, through the payment of speaker, conference, and research fees that functioned as kickbacks.

The suit references twenty examples of Novo Nordisk sponsoring studies, seminars, trips, meals, and honoraria for army physicians from 2005 to 2007. Ian Black cited, as an example, that in 2005 the company paid army physicians to attend an anesthesiology board meeting in Atlanta. Black and other physicians were driven around in limos, put up at the Ritz-Carlton, and given meals at New York Prime, a four-star steakhouse, and Emeril's, another high-end restaurant. Novo Nordisk's sales representatives were similarly rewarded, according to the suit. They were given, for example, a trip on the *Queen Elizabeth 2* to visit Novo Nordisk's collection of castles in Denmark.

It is, however, illegal for a company outside the government to pay inducements to federal employees. Army physicians are required to follow federal laws and military regulations that generally prohibit honoraria and many types of gifts from third parties. In order to hide those payments, the lawsuit alleged, Novo Nordisk funded the "TRUE Research Foundation for the Advancement of Military Medicine," which functioned as a "money-laundering device through which Novo [Nordisk] funneled cash to military doctors willing to promote the use of [Factor Seven] to their colleagues." Novo Nordisk indeed later admitted that they had made payments to the T.R.U.E. foundation, which was based in San Antonio not far from the Institute of Surgical Research. The lawsuit goes on to describe the T.R.U.E. foundation as a "sham" organization.

Indeed the initials in the T.R.U.E. acronym didn't actually stand for anything. The executive director of the foundation wanted to call the organization True Research Foundation but discovered that there was another entity that had a similar name. Her lawyers suggested placing periods after each letter in the word *TRUE*. The foundation's research director explained the activities of the organization in the following way: "If a military doctor had to go present findings for his research, we could pay for his travel to go present the findings. If he wanted to hire (someone) to come in to help him with his research, we would hire him a body. Hell, if they needed a new computer, we could buy them a new computer." Novo Nordisk denied any wrongdoing, arguing that it was perfectly legal for the organization to take donations from pharmaceutical companies and others and to work independently with the military to fund medical studies.

While the *United States v. Novo Nordisk* lawsuit was under review, on a sunny spring day in 2010 an enterprising reporter from the *San Antonio Express-News* went to the T.R.U.E. Research Foundation's headquarters, which was in Suite 705 of Energy Plaza, a modernist office complex at 8610 North New Braunfels Avenue. There, the reporter discovered a federal investigator, wearing a dark suit and who appeared to be in his thirties, entering the offices of Terri Nakamura. He said he was from the Department of Justice and was looking into Novo Nordisk. The investigator wanted check stubs and other financial documents. He returned at least two more times.

Public documents revealed that significant amounts of money passed through the T.R.U.E. Research Foundation. In 2009 the gross receipts of the T.R.U.E. foundation, whose stated mission was "improving the quality of military medicine through research and education," were about $13 million. The executive director of the foundation was Jean Bordas, whose annual compensation was about $230,000. She appeared to have no formal scientific credentials to justify the position. Terri Nakamura, the research director, was Bordas's daughter and also appeared not to have relevant credentials. It was later reported by the *San Antonio Express-News* that Bordas and Nakamura frequently clashed and that the foundation's board was unhappy with their spending habits.

The federal whistleblower investigation continued on for another full year, almost three years after Black and Montiel filed their suit. In their long and no doubt agonizing waiting game for an answer, it may have been a foreboding sign that in 2010 the FDA added a warning to the label of Factor Seven, stating that the drug could cause unwanted and potentially deadly blood clots in arteries when given to non-hemophiliacs.

Notably the alert was placed in a "black box," which is reserved for the FDA's highest and most stringent safety warning.

CHAPTER ELEVEN

The Army's Greatest Invention

IN THE FALL of 2008, just as Ian Black and Oscar Montiel filed their federal suit, Bart was stopped at a red light in his new maroon Lexus in Tequesta, Florida—a town just north of Palm Beach. He had just dropped off Sarah, who was now thirteen, at her private middle school. On the drive there, Bart had put on a good front for Sarah, as he always did, trying to give no indication that he was depressed. But in truth she knew exactly what was going on and it impacted her greatly. He was in the middle of the period of breakdown, and he felt bruised and angry from the moment he woke up to the time he went to bed. The fight with the army and Holcomb was at an impasse, and he had not reconciled with Frank. Nonetheless he was still collecting a very sizable salary and advising On-Site Gas and Z-Medica from afar.

When he bought the SUV, he had instructed the car dealer to install a custom Florida license plate that read "QUIKCLT." As Bart sat at the red light, feeling numb and empty, an old pickup truck pulled up in the lane next to him. The driver, a middle-aged and rather grizzled-looking man, rolled down his passenger-side window and shouted over at Bart, "Hey!! Did you have anything to do with QuikClot??"

Bart shouted back, "Yes. I helped invent it!"

"That stuff saved my son's life in Iraq!" the man bellowed. "God bless you!"

Bart was trying to formulate some kind of response when the light turned green. The man drove off, waving back at Bart, then giving him a thumbs-up out the window, an eternal gesture of gratitude.

It was not long after this encounter that Bart and Linda agreed to file for divorce. They did so with heavy hearts and a deep, mutual sadness. Bart had hoped that the decision to split up would be accompanied by a release of psychic pressure, but it did not. Instead it just drove home his sense of failure as a husband and father. After the separation, Bart moved out of the house and into a recreational vehicle that had sleeping and cooking accommodations, which he kept in an RV park in Juno Beach, four miles away from the house in Palm Beach Gardens. He spent his days largely wandering around, shocked at all that had transpired in the past couple of years. Once again he took up golf, but he found that PGA-level courses in Florida were beyond his skill level. He bought a $20,000 Orange County chopper motorcycle but hardly rode it. He called it his "death wish made visible," and sold it six months later. He walked five miles a day, and spent hours driving around aimlessly, eating fast food. He also took his boat out and fished. Bart did almost all of this alone, as he had few friends in Florida, having moved there only fairly recently. By far his happiest moments during that time were on the days when he went snorkeling at an inlet under a bridge, where he swam through a wonderland of tropical fish. It was only there could he find escape.

Five months later he bought a condo, where he lived alone, along the Intracoastal Waterway.

He did some work for Frank during this time, but not much. Frank was now thinking that Bart had essentially gone crazy. Still, Bart was concerned when he saw that both businesses, On-Site Gas and Z-Medica, had stagnated in his absence. The divorce from Linda became finalized in a matter of months, primarily because Bart and his attorney chose not to contest Linda's request for a sizable amount of alimony. He still loved Linda and wanted her to be comfortable. When Bart signed the papers in court without negotiating any of its terms, the judge said that in all his years on the bench he had never seen a divorce case proceed so smoothly. Over the following years, Bart would support Linda substantially far beyond what he was required to do by the terms of the agreement.

In 2008, Bart moved out of the Florida house and returned to Connecticut. For many months he lived out of a suitcase in a Courtyard by Marriott hotel in Cromwell, a suburban town equidistant between the offices of Z-Medica and On-Site Gas. He got his coffee every morning from a Dunkin' Donuts a block from the highway and ate at diners. But slowly, he was beginning to feel that he could function again, or at least pretend to. It was like coming out of a years-long stupor. He met with Frank, and they agreed that Bart would gradually return to the office, attending meetings and managing sales strategies for both companies. Still, Bart sensed that Frank was a little gun-shy about his return, wondering if Bart would maintain his stability.

Bart and Frank both also arrived at the conclusion that they needed to fire Steven. Frank had initially been impressed by Steven's credentials but now saw how deeply he had impacted morale at Z-Medica. And of course Steven had been obstructionist to Bart, all but shutting him out of the business as much as he could. But now Bart was back. Frank and Bart met with Steven and placed a sizable check in front of him. He could either take the check and leave or be fired. He took the check, and Bart and Frank never saw him again.

As Bart slowly got back up to speed, he realized how much he had missed while he was away. In Florida he had been under the impression that he knew what was going on at Z-Medica, but he had been wrong. Frank and Steven had been working on a new formulation of QuikClot, one that wouldn't cause burns. Frank knew that they would have to find a new mineral to form its base. This new mineral—should one even exist—would have to have the same capacity to clot blood, while, and this was critical, not emitting any heat. Ideally it would also be possible to impregnate the material into gauze so the product could be applied easily, cleanly, and efficiently. *But did such a rock or mineral actually exist?* It seemed unlikely. Frank's paradigm-shifting discovery had been out in the world for six years now, and no scientists or medical or drug companies had found any other agent or mineral that could do what zeolite was capable of.

But in his quiet, unassuming, and deeply intuitive way, Frank had already—four years earlier—identified a mineral called kaolin as a potential replacement. Characteristically, he hadn't discussed the hemostatic properties of kaolin with anyone, not even Bart, and had mentioned them only briefly in an obscure patent application that he had written in 2004. One of the most commonly mined products in the world, kaolin is a soft, chalky mineral, typically white or yellow. In the United States, kaolin is heavily mined in central Georgia, so much so that the stretch between Augusta and Macon is sometimes called "the white gold belt." Kaolin is safe when introduced into the human body; in fact, the common over-the-counter antidiarrheal agent Kaopectate contains kaolin. Since the early 1950s, kaolin has been used in what is called the kaolin clotting test (KCT), a blood test to check for antibodies that cause a blood clotting disorder. Kaolin and calcium are added to blood samples, and the time it takes for a clot to form is measured.

Given that the KCT has long been a standard lab test in medicine, it was strange that no one had investigated kaolin's capacity to clot blood when directly introduced into the bloodstream. Frank, in fact, knew nothing about the KCT test. But with the same depth of insight that had led him to envision the blood clotting properties of zeolite, Frank somehow intuited that kaolin might have the same potential. In a patent application that he wrote on December 2, 2004, Frank proposed that the loose granules of zeolite in QuikClot, so they wouldn't spill messily into the wound, be put in a binder of clay, which would function as an alternate delivery system and enhance the clotting properties of his original invention. He identified kaolin as a potential material for the binder. Frank wrote:

> The binder is preferably clay-based and may further include fillers (e.g., aluminum sulfate) or thickening agents that facilitate the selective application of the zeolite in various forms....Natural clays that may provide suitable bases include, but are not limited to, kaolin, kaolinite, bentonite, montmorillonite, combinations of the foregoing clays, and the like.

As usual Frank was working entirely alone. As was often the case with Frank's proposals, the details were rather unclear. Frank didn't explain why kaolin would work as a binder or how it would help facilitate the clotting of blood, or even much about what the binder would look like. But his thinking, commonsensical yet elegant as ever, was as follows: If zeolite, a cheap and natural mineral, absorbed the water in blood, who was to say there wasn't another mineral that could do the same thing? The principle would be the same: caverns in a mineral would soak things up like a sponge.

But unlike with zeolite, Frank had no hands-on experience with kaolin. He needed the expertise of a true mineral scientist. Once again, Michael Given and Joe Dacorta turned to Galen Stucky, the University of California chemist, who had previously worked on the silver-enhanced versions of QuikClot. With funding from the Office of Naval Research, whose role would prove absolutely essential to the success of what was about to transpire, Stucky assembled a small team of graduate students to investigate the hemostatic properties of kaolin. They tested kaolin against the original granular QuikClot and discovered that it worked just as well, but without any of the large heat release. Frank of course was delighted to hear this. This finding could be the game changer he was looking for, one that would forever dismiss the Achilles' heel of the original QuikClot that it could burn soldiers. Stucky and his students also happily found that when introduced into the area of an injury, the nanoparticles of kaolin congregated at the wound site and did not enter the circulatory system. Furthermore, the talc-like quality and texture of kaolin meant it lent itself perfectly to being impregnated into standard gauze.

With great speed—in less than two weeks—Stucky and his team created a prototype of the product. They added the kaolin to gauze strips three inches wide and twelve feet long and folded the pieces, rather than placing them on a roll, as is typical. Remarkably, a twelve-foot-long sheet of the gauze fit into a single packet. The product had a five-year shelf life and cost thirty-three dollars a package, which made it more expensive than the original zeolite version but still far cheaper than HemCon. The prototype was used on a trial basis by special forces personnel and the Coast Guard. Tests of the gauze by the Israel Defense Force's Medical Corps showed an approximate 90 percent effectiveness in stopping hemorrhage. The navy and Marine Corps then gave Z-Medica almost $3 million to conduct human studies of the kaolin product at Johns Hopkins, the University of Miami, the University of Massachusetts Medical School, Vanderbilt University, and Hartford Hospital. The investigations would determine kaolin gauze's ability to stop bleeding in high-velocity bullet wounds and battlefield injuries. It all seemed too good to be true, but it wasn't. It was as if, all of a sudden, after six years on the periphery, Z-Medica had arrived at the center of the military and medical establishment.

Bart was astounded to learn the details of this progress upon his return, and a little embarrassed by how little he had been a part of it. But now that he was functioning better than he had in years, he inserted himself into the final steps of the development of the kaolin product just as he had done with QuikClot six years before. Bart negotiated a payment to Stucky for his contribution and intellectual property, writing him a check for more than $1 million. To the consternation of some on the team, Bart, now acting like his old self, got involved with the naming of the new product halfway through the process. The team had already come up with the straightforward name "Combat Gauze," with no additions or modifications. But Bart insisted that the name must also include the word "QuikClot" so that the new gauze would be seen as part of the QuikClot family of products. "Whatever one thought of QuikClot," he argued, "it worked. By identifying the new product with QuikClot, we are buying instant credibility." Hence "QuikClot Combat Gauze" was born and put on the market in early 2008. It completely replaced the zeolite form of QuikClot, which Z-Medica stopped making.

Yet another pivotal development occurred when the US military, with the army at the forefront, officially stated that QuikClot Combat Gauze, based on its incontrovertible efficacy, was better than HemCon. This was the breakthrough Bart and Frank had been waiting for for years. In April 2008 the Committee on Tactical Combat Casualty Care, the group that sets protocol and recommendations for military trauma medicine, recommended "Combat Gauze as the first-line treatment for life-threatening hemorrhage that is not amenable to tourniquet placement." To his credit, it was John Holcomb who made the formal recommendation. It was one of his last official acts as director of the Institute of Surgical Research. This meant that all soldiers, in every service branch, would have Combat Gauze in their first-aid kits. It was an almost unimaginable victory. Tiny Z-Medica had defeated the US Army and all the products, specifically Factor Seven and HemCon, that it had backed. The designation by the committee effectively sounded the death knell for the HemCon company, and its profits dried up almost overnight.

When the news came through, Bart was back in Florida, finishing up some business with Linda. But once back in Connecticut, he and Frank met to celebrate. Awkwardly, they raised glasses of champagne in Frank's office at On-Site. Bart was ebullient, and Frank clearly satisfied but characteristically muted. He said what he always said whenever there was good news: "Well, that's pretty good, isn't it?"

After the endorsement of Combat Gauze by all military branches, orders for the product were voluminous. The army alone bought 270,000 packages of Combat Gauze, and the other service branches bought hundreds of thousands of units. Orders came in from all over the world: Canada, Britain, Australia, France, Mexico. Within a year, Z-Medica sold 3.5 million bandages. The company scaled up to three shifts a day—its staff worked around the clock, and for a while they still couldn't meet demand. Bart hired dozens more workers, often friends and relatives of existing staff. The war in Iraq was still fierce, and Bart told each new employee, "Every order we don't fill means that someone could lose their life. We aren't primarily in the business of making money; we are in the business of saving lives!" He would repeat the sentiment every time he visited the factory floor.

In August 2008, at the annual military medical conference, Galen Stucky won the Department of Defense's Advanced Technology Applications for Combat Casualty Care Award for his contributions to the development of Combat Gauze. Stucky said, "I am very honored. In retrospect, this project has meant more to me than any other I've worked on for the past forty years."

And then a final remarkable, if nefarious, event occurred. In a press release dated September 18, 2009, the army claimed credit for the invention of Combat Gauze. The statement was entitled "U.S. Army Recognizes Top Ten Greatest Inventions of 2008," and it listed "inventions that were fielded within the Army during 2008." At number seven on the list was Combat Gauze. Its developer was identified as "U.S. Army Institute of Surgical Research," and Z-Medica was not mentioned at all.

Everyone at Z-Medica, including Frank, was livid. Even mild-mannered Michael Given at the Office of Naval Research demanded a retraction. "How could they even do this?" Frank asked. It was as if their achievement and sacrifice had been stolen from them. Bart's answer to the question was simple and emphatic. "They can do whatever they want. They are the US Army. They have the money and power, but we alone have the truth." In fact, Bart, ever the marketer, viewed this as *the* moment of ultimate triumph. He barged into Frank's office. He was so charged up he was almost shouting. He couldn't contain himself. "Frank, we've won!! Now that the army has claimed credit for Combat Gauze, they won't ever come after us again. It would be like attacking themselves! For all I care, John Holcomb can win fifty awards for saying he invented it." Frank struggled to grasp this fully. He smiled awkwardly. "Don't you get it, Frank?" Bart said. "We've won. We have fucking won!"

Frank thought about it a moment. "Yeah, I guess we did," he said.

Bart and Frank appeared to have won even more when, a few months after Combat Gauze's victory, they finally heard about John Holcomb's resignation from the Institute of Surgical Research. One would think that Bart in particular would have been ebullient and celebratory. But actually he wasn't. Now that Combat Gauze had been named the recommended hemostatic agent of the entire military, Holcomb didn't matter that much anymore.

Either way, Bart found himself feeling better than he had in years.

It took almost three years from the time of the original filing, but on June 10, 2011, the United States Department of Justice announced that Novo Nordisk had settled with the government, agreeing to pay $25 million to resolve its civil liability arising from the illegal promotion of Factor Seven. Black and Montiel received about $3.5 million each. The Department of Justice's press release stated that "the Department of Defense was influenced by Novo's unlawful off-label promotion and purchased NovoSeven to treat service members wounded in Iraq and Afghanistan.... While Novo Nordisk admitted no liability as part of the settlement, it did agree to enter into an expansive corporate integrity agreement with the Office of the Attorney General of the Department of Health and Human Services. That agreement provides for procedures and reviews to be put in place to avoid... conduct similar to that which gave rise to this matter." Unsurprisingly, almost concurrent to the lawsuit's resolution, the T.R.U.E. Research Foundation ceased operations and then filed for bankruptcy in June 2011.

But given that Novo Nordisk had been transformed into a

blockbuster drug in the period covered by the allegations, the amount of the settlement seems rather trivial. "You couldn't get a more graphic example of why there should be much more criminal prosecutions of companies like this," said Dr. Sidney Wolfe of the consumer rights advocacy group Public Citizen. "They got off easy in terms of the amount of money they paid and no one went to jail."

Ian Black left the military and set up a medical practice in Vermont. Oscar Montiel left medical sales and opened a restaurant in San Antonio. Later, Black told a San Antonio newspaper how he was seduced by Novo Nordisk. "It's all hindsight, but they were so shrewd. It was brilliant because you had all these young physicians," Black said. "[These doctors] had no research background. It's not like they had been in a research lab for years and years…'Do you want to talk about your experience?' 'Sure. You're going to fly me where, to Las Vegas or down to Atlanta and I get to eat in Emeril's restaurant? Wow.'…You know, I was wined and dined by the companies and it was flattering, and I thought I was cutting edge and whatnot."

In the aftermath of the settlement, Ian Black said, "I wasn't trying to assign blame or to make money, I just wanted it to stop." Black said about his time serving wounded soldiers, "I am proud of the care we gave. I know to a man we did, and would have done, anything to help those soldiers. Maybe that was the problem, that eagerness to help. I look back and I wonder, Did I hurt someone?"

———————

Meanwhile, John Holcomb appeared to have won too. He maintained his high profile at the University of Texas at Austin medical school. In 2011 he was a spokesperson of the care team of Congresswoman Gabby Giffords when she was transferred to the Memorial Hermann-Texas Medical Center for a lengthy rehabilitation after being shot eight times in a parking lot in Tucson. Ironically, Combat Gauze had been used on some of the other eighteen victims of the shooting. Holcomb also began collecting accolades for his military service. In 2009, Holcomb's successor at the Institute of Surgical Research, along with his predecessor, Basil Pruitt, wrote a tribute in the *Journal of Trauma* about his leadership at the institute. The article was entitled "The Warrior's Combat Surgeon" and featured a picture of a very young and rugged-looking Holcomb in camo army gear in Mogadishu. They wrote, "John Holcomb's six years of leadership at the...helm were transformational.... He brought tourniquets to every deployed US soldier, airman, sailor, and marine in the combat zone. He ushered in a new era of wound management by deploying the first hemostatic dressings in recorded history—abruptly modernizing thousands of years of cloth wound dressings. Many service members will be coming home to the ones they love and who love them—all because of the untiring passion of John Holcomb to improve combat casualty care." In 2011 former army surgeon General James Peake said about Holcomb, "All he cared about was doing what was right by the soldiers and stopping bleeding." In 2014, Holcomb won the Major Jonathan Letterman Medical Excellence Award from the National Museum of Civil War Medicine for his achievement in battlefield medicine. In 2017, the military news website Special Operations Forces Report wrote, "There is no one who has been responsible for saving more lives among U.S. casualties in Iraq and Afghanistan than John Holcomb."

But his legacy is far more complicated than that. If one examines the scorecard of the products and innovations that Holcomb backed, the results are sobering. The fibrin bandage with the American Red Cross failed. HemCon ultimately failed. Factor Seven failed. PolyHeme, a controversial blood substitute that Holcomb championed, failed.

But there is another side of the ledger. At the Institute of Surgical Research, Holcomb led the design of a trauma registry system that coordinated and organized battlefield medical care. He played a crucial role in the successful revamping of transportation systems that brought the wounded to appropriate levels of care, which involved a complex collaboration among frontline units, forward surgical teams, and hospitals. Holcomb's support for tourniquets was an unqualified success. Here his doggedness and resolute willingness to go against the tide undoubtedly saved many lives. Perhaps Holcomb's daring and his failures cannot be truly separated from each other. Historians and observers of the medical innovations of war focus almost solely on the breakthroughs and overlook the many missteps. Holcomb's track record may not be so very different from that of other battlefield pioneers.

One of Holcomb's innovations is still under debate. During the Battle of Mogadishu, Holcomb's surgical team was supplied with frozen blood plasma to be used for transfusions. In the dire conditions, a number of the bags unexpectedly broke, which left Holcomb without access to platelets and plasma. In desperation, he and his colleagues drew blood from volunteers in the hospital, which they then transfused into some of the wounded soldiers. "We were all young surgeons and we were doing what we thought was crazy," Holcomb said. But later, Holcomb realized that the patients who were transfused directly with the whole blood from volunteers seemed to fare better than soldiers given transfusions of the component parts of blood.

At the time that Holcomb served in Mogadishu, the transfusing of whole blood had completely fallen out of favor in trauma care. It was a relic of an earlier generation, one from before the 1960s and the advent of polyvinyl containers and sterilized tubes, which allow the components of blood to be stored as separate products: red blood cells, plasma, and platelets. Being able to store these components separately ushered in what was called component therapy, which allowed for bleeding patients to be given only the components they needed most. Component therapy was considered a state-of-the-art, major advance, despite somewhat limited data on its effectiveness. From the Vietnam War era onward, transfusing whole blood occurred only in austere environments such as developing countries and far-flung military field hospitals, as occurred with Holcomb in Mogadishu.

But after Mogadishu, Holcomb argued that component therapy had practical disadvantages. He wrote, "Blood banks and bedside clinicians all report difficulty with coordinating the preparation, thawing, checking, delivering, and transfusing all these products at the same time and in the correct order." Part of the difficulty arises from the fact that each component has a different shelf life, making it hard to keep track of them. Holcomb asserted that "time lost coordinating the different blood components could have enormous consequences on outcomes." In massively bleeding patients, he argued, every minute counts.

At the start of the wars in Iraq and Afghanistan, the US military was fundamentally opposed to whole blood for fear that it would lead to contamination and infection. The guidelines indicated the following:

Field conditions are inherently unsanitary and are presumed to increase the risk of bacterial contamination of the blood. . . . It is NOT appropriate, as a matter of convenience, to use FWB [fresh whole blood] as an alternative to more stringently controlled blood products for patients who do not have severe, immediately life-threatening injuries.

But as the war wore on in Afghanistan, separated blood components were not always available. Platelets in particular were often in short supply. Safety concerns were now less of a concern: soldiers were screened for infectious diseases before deployment and freshly drawn blood was tested for HIV and syphilis. Once again the army began using whole blood. Since then, emerging research, some done by Holcomb, has shown promising, if still not conclusive, results. It is quite likely that whole blood transfusions would not have been reevaluated without Holcomb's obstinacy.

But the legacy of Factor Seven, and its impact on the lives and deaths of soldiers, is no less than an American tragedy. In retrospect, it is evident that the aggressive promotion of Factor Seven beyond its intended and approved use and into the arms of thousands of army soldiers transpired on the very margins of acceptable medicine. The conditions that brought Factor Seven to soldiers like Caleb Lufkin and Shane Mahaffee were the outcome of the highly dangerous, potentially fatal collision of the arrogance, massive budgets, and unchecked power structure of army medicine; the extreme profitability of pharmaceutical companies; and the lack of regulation of off-label use of medication. The vast amounts of money involved—too much of it, and too much lust for it—is the one thing that connects all three of these factors. Additionally, within the field of trauma medicine, an emotion-driven culture—which gave rise to the use of Factor Seven, rather than considered and evidence-based practices for traumatic bleeding—continues unabated. Ian Roberts, the English epidemiologist and expert on bleeding disorders, said, "When that amount of money is exposed to science and medicine, particularly military medicine, things like evidence get distorted. Money makes the research enterprise sort of like a fun house or kaleidoscope, filled with crazy mirrors." Roberts adds that trauma doctors and researchers continue to function in exactly the wrong way. "They have enthusiasm for an intervention, and they do the clinical trial," Roberts says. "They should do the clinical trial, and if the results are good, then they should have enthusiasm."

A kind of inverse proof of the distorting power of money in trauma medicine can be found in the story of tranexamic acid. Tranexamic acid, which helps the body from prematurely breaking down blood clots, is an effective treatment for traumatic bleeding. An international research team did a study in 2010 on twenty thousand trauma patients in forty countries and found that tranexamic acid decreased mortality by about 10 percent compared with placebo. It is estimated that the drug could save up to 128,000 of those lives a year, four thousand of them in the United States. Tranexamic acid has since been incorporated into American and British military protocols, and has been named by the World Health Organization as an essential drug. But because tranexamic acid—which is a generic drug—is so cheap the treatment has never fully taken off. As the *New York Times* wrote in 2012: "the drug's very inexpensiveness has slowed its entry into American emergency rooms...Because there is so little profit in it, the companies that make it do not champion it."

The conditions that created the aggressive and copious use of Factor Seven by the military seem unchanged. For one thing, Novo Nordisk continues its aggressive tactics. Some years after the settlement with the Department of Justice, a second whistleblower case against Novo Nordisk for Factor Seven is currently underway in the United States District Court for the Western District of Oklahoma and has yet to be resolved. The Siegel case, so called because its whistleblower is a Dr. Jamie Siegel, bears striking resemblances to Montiel and Black's lawsuit. Dr. Siegel is a specialist in oncology and hematology. In 2008 she became the director of hematology in Clinical Development, Medical and Regulatory Affairs at Novo Nordisk. She expected her work to revolve around developing clinical trials and research but came to believe that the company focused on marketing at the expense of such developments. She left Novo Nordisk in 2009.

First filed in 2015 and sealed until 2020, Siegel's lawsuit accuses Novo Nordisk of attempting to increase profits from using Factor Seven on a small subgroup of hemophilia patients by promoting the drug for off-label uses in a manner that minimized the drug's safety risks. Dr. Siegel's allegations relate to the population for which Ulla Hedner invented Factor Seven: hemophiliacs with inhibitors. Factor Seven was FDA approved to be taken by patients with inhibitors on an as-needed basis, but the complaint alleges that the company promoted the off-label use of taking the drug daily, as a prophylactic. The case also alleges that Novo Nordisk paid kickbacks to "anyone who could influence" the prescribing of Factor Seven—including the patient, their family, the physician, and pharmacies. Siegel's case paints a picture of Novo Nordisk continuing to double down on aggressive marketing toward hemophilia patients even after the Montiel and Black settlement. Novo Nordisk denies any wrongdoing, and the case is ongoing in federal court. A judge has not yet ruled on the matter.

Additionally, Novo Nordisk has recently had to pay a large settlement for ethical violations with another drug. In 2017, Novo Nordisk paid a settlement of $58 million for failure to comply with FDA rules in the marketing of the diabetes drug Victoza. One of the potential risks of Victoza is a rare form of cancer, medullary thyroid carcinoma, and the FDA required that Novo Nordisk inform physicians of this risk. According to the Department of Justice, however, "some Novo Nordisk sales representatives gave information to physicians that created the false or misleading impression that the [FDA-required] message was erroneous, irrelevant, or unimportant."

The US Congress has also investigated apparent collusion around price increases for insulin products made by three competing companies, including Novo Nordisk. The three companies control 90 percent of the market for insulin. The investigation noted thirteen occasions in which the prices of Sanofi and Novo Nordisk insulin products rose in lockstep. Novo Nordisk also raised the price of the insulin product NovoLog by 627 percent since its launch. Shareholders took Novo Nordisk to court in Denmark, demanding that it pay the equivalent of $1.8 billion for not properly disclosing its United States insulin profits. The case was settled in 2022, though with no admission of liability or payments to plaintiffs by Novo Nordisk.

In the wake of the Factor Seven lawsuit and other controversies around off-label marketing and prescribing practices, there have been calls for more monitoring of these practices by the FDA. A recent review of off-label prescribing among office-based physicians found that 73 percent of off-label prescribing had little or no scientific support. The FDA's system of reporting adverse events has also been criticized. Currently, the reporting of adverse events is not mandated, but done on a voluntary basis, leading to vast underreporting.

All this is to say that Novo Nordisk appears to be continuing its aggressive strategies, and no meaningful regulatory changes have occurred in the last decade. The conditions that created the American tragedy of Factor Seven remain the same, which of course allows for a similar episode to occur in the future.

And finally, as to the question of whether the US Army has changed: when the administrative investigative unit of the army was contacted for the full records regarding the army's investigation into John Holcomb and his colleagues and their exact relationships with Novo Nordisk, this was its response, a masterpiece of bureaucratic equivocation (note that the memo refers to Factor Seven by its consumer name, NovoSeven):

The Staff Judge Advocates Office (OSJA) has purview over Administrative Investigations, which includes Command Inquiries and Investigations. At the time of this investigation, Army Regulation 15-6, Procedures for Administrative Investigations and Boards of Officers, did not include a requirement to store records. However, it was the practice of the Medical Command OSJA office to store copies of the 15-6 investigations for five years. A records search for the AR 15-6 investigation pertaining to any Command inquiry/Investigation related to the use of the drug Novoseven and the receipt of honoraria for related medical research by doctors at the Army Institute for Surgical Research was conducted by the Staff Judge Advocate's Office, Office of the Surgeon General/Headquarters, U.S. Army Medical Command.

Additionally, the Headquarters, U.S. Army Medical Command Staff Judge Advocate Office directed that a search for records also be conducted by the Staff Judge Advocate Office of the U.S. Army Medical Research and Material Command and by the Command Judge Advocate Office of Brooke Army Medical Center, Joint Base San Antonio, Fort Sam Houston, TX. After making a good faith effort and conducting a thorough search of records using methods which can reasonably be expected to produce the information requested, an AR 15-6 report of investigation related to the use of the drug Novoseven and the receipt of Honoria [sic] as specified in your request could not be located.

When it came to the United States Army, the system covered up its tracks, preventing full and final answers. In other words, the prevailing system endured, with no recognition, or even apparent awareness, of its failings.

The Left Side of the Menu

Everything in my life was merely prologue until now.
—André Aciman, *Find Me*

IN THE YEARS after being deployed in Iraq, Tim Coakley experienced significant depressions as well as symptoms of post-traumatic stress disorder, along with traumatic brain injuries from repeated exposure to explosives. Even though he still functioned as a high-ranking navy officer and medical doctor, rising to the rank of commander, his sense of self-worth and confidence were decimated over the years. He could never—and still cannot—understand why his lived experience of using QuikClot in combat was questioned and devalued by higher-ups in the army. After his divorce, his personal life was in tatters, although he remained devoted to his five children and later his three grandchildren. He underwent intensive individual and group psychotherapy as well as cognitive and occupational therapy to help rewire his brain after the neurological traumas he suffered. The turning point in his recovery occurred in 2008 when he became the deputy force surgeon for the Navy Expeditionary Combat Command in Virginia Beach, which gave him medical oversight of 47,000 sailors. But given his taste for adventure and his complete inability to say no to assignments, he ended up undertaking numerous special missions for the navy and marines between 2009 and 2011. The details of some of these missions remain classified. But he treated villagers in the depths of the Amazon, taught hyperbaric medicine to members of the Brazilian armed forces, and assisted in the rescue of dozens of Somali refugees who were starving on a raft in the Indian Ocean. He treated one woman on the raft who was on the verge of giving birth and got her safely to a hospital in Kuwait, where she delivered a healthy child.

In 2011, Coakley was named a member of the steering committee of the Recovering Warrior Task Force for the Department of Defense, in which capacity he helped set best practices for the treatment of traumatic brain injury and post-traumatic stress disorder. Given his own history, this was a special honor for Coakley. He retired from the navy in 2011 and became medical director of emergency medical services for a large hospital system in Virginia. Now he is much in demand as an emergency medicine and trauma medicine consultant and trainer, and he was recently involved in delivering hundreds of thousands of medical supply units, including Combat Gauze, to Ukraine. In addition, he has started his own emergency medicine consulting firm that has received federal contracts and operates internationally. But for all his accomplishments, he still suffers nightmares and flashbacks. It is only in the last year that he has been able to once again enter into a long-term relationship, his first in years.

For his part, Joe Dacorta too left the navy, in his case not long after the controversies and conflict around QuikClot and HemCon, and partially because of his embitterment about the army's resistance to the product. He went on to hold senior positions in product development for medical companies, most of which supplied products to the military. Recently retired, he lives in suburban Virginia with his wife, a designer, and takes great pride in the thriving careers of his three daughters, who are writers and artists. Even in retirement he has written six patents for innovations in medical devices and pharmaceuticals. He also takes care of his two dogs, goes on long walks, sails up and down the East Coast in the summers, and reads books—ranging from the philosophy of science to poetry to works of history—at night. He is proud of his legacy in the navy, one that brought him to some of the most obscure and dangerous corners of the world, but he is equally happy to leave all the politics of the military behind. Now in his late sixties, he still seems slightly staggered by how the army fought against QuikClot so aggressively. He remains angry, saying, "I just never thought they would go that low. We were just ordinary people in extraordinary circumstances, but we had a product that was saving lives." He sees Bart and Frank and the Z-Medica team as entirely unique in their level of resolve. "Almost every other contractor would have given up when the army came after them. Z-Medica was literally the one in a thousand that wouldn't stop."

Dacorta and Coakley, who became good friends, remain united in their devotion to Tom Eagles, or Tommy, as they still call him. Eagles died on June 3, 2016, in South Carolina at age seventy-one due to complications from Agent Orange exposure as well as all the bullets he took "in the ass," as he said, in Vietnam. His obituary notice is filled with moving tributes to his service, many of the messages seeming to tell the story of the Vietnam War in miniature. One entry says, "Doc, you got point man this time—REST EASY MY FRIEND—thanks for patching me up in '67 when I took the hit." As illustrious and colorful as his career was—he remains by all accounts the most decorated medic in American military history—he counted the adoption of QuikClot, or "fairy dust," as he sometimes called it, as one of his greatest achievements. At his retirement dinner, Bart was a guest of honor, sitting next to Eagles and across from General Peter Pace, now chairman of the Joint Chiefs of Staff, who had signed the letter that sprang QuikClot into the world.

––––––––––

In the summer and early fall of 2012, Bart Gullong was once again living out of an RV, now in Old Saybrook, Connecticut. The RV—a thirty-six-foot-long Winnebago Journey—had been nicknamed "the big brown rolling turd" by his daughter. He had recently sold his home in Florida and been living in the turd for three months, stationed in a back corner of the parking lot of the Island Cove Marina, where it was hooked up to electrical power and running water.

On a Friday afternoon in September, Bart received a telephone call from his attorney, a call that he'd been anticipating for some time. In a certain way he had been waiting his whole life for this phone call. The attorney said that there was a check waiting for Bart at his office, five miles away. Bart immediately drove his car to the office, picked up the envelope, and then sped to the Bank of America branch in town before it closed. His hand trembled slightly as he wrote in the amount of the deposit on the bank slip. There were many integers involved, so many that he almost ran out of space on the appointed line. As he walked up to the teller, Bart wondered if she would show any reaction when she saw the amount of the deposit. But the teller revealed nothing, processing the transaction and giving Bart a receipt in the same cool manner with which bank tellers typically operate.

Receipt in hand, Bart strolled back to his car. He climbed in, shut the door, and then pounded the steering wheel. He then lifted his head skyward and howled with joy and satisfaction. Outside of the birth of Sarah, it was a depth of joy and satisfaction that he had never felt before. But the elation wasn't just about the money; it was also the indescribable satisfaction of the recognition that he had succeeded at doing something good for the world, which was the goal that he had set for himself in his hippieish days at Marietta College.

In the last three years, after QuikClot Combat Gauze entered the market, Bart and Frank had experienced for the first time in their careers one success after another. Combat Gauze, with its demonstrated effectiveness, ease of use, and complete lack of an exothermic reaction, simply proved unstoppable. Its acceptance by all military branches led to millions of orders after the product's introduction. Furthermore, the US military's backing of Combat Gauze as its official "hemostatic agent of choice" led to orders flooding in from militaries all over the world, as well as from police departments and first responders from every corner of the globe. Z-Medica's staff tripled almost overnight, and three shifts needed to work twenty-four hours a day out of the Wallingford office to fill the rush of orders. Z-Medica also developed a less potent consumer version, available on Amazon.com and at Walmart and sporting goods stores everywhere. Soon enough, Combat Gauze had thousands of reviews on Amazon, with an average rating of 4.8 out of 5. A typical review read:

5.0 out of 5 stars **These are life savers for major bleeding.**
Strongly recommended by medical personnel the world over. These kaolin-based clotting gauze are an essential item for everyone's home, car and sports of every kind. These + a professional tourniquet can mean the difference between life and death.

The one area that Bart and his growing team continued to have difficulties reaching, however, was the hospital market. In theory, there was nothing to prevent the use of Combat Gauze to stanch bleeding after surgeries in the operating room, but doctors seemed reluctant to adopt a product they associated with first aid and the first responder market, which was somehow deemed not sufficiently "clinical" or "medical." Despite Combat Gauze's unassailable efficacy, the stubbornly conservative medical establishment continued to look down on the product. Also, as a practical matter, the Z-Medica marketing staff found it difficult to access the decision makers at hospitals. Bulk purchasing orders were made by impenetrable committees that did not want to speak directly to vendors and, even when they did, often took years to make a decision. Despite the fact that Z-Medica had now hired well-qualified physicians as medical directors, doctors were often too busy and distracted to talk to them, still thinking of Z-Medica as "down market" and not a fully legitimate medical supplier.

But in every other area, Combat Gauze was in high demand—among the leaders in the global hemostatic agent market. Soon enough, Z-Medica was approached by numerous private equity groups, most of them specializing in buyouts of midsize health-care companies. Frank and Bart, after much discussion, decided they might be interested in selling. As Bart always said, he was more interested in, and better at, building the airplane than actually keeping it flying. Besides, Bart was now sixty-four and Frank almost seventy.

They received bids from numerous equity firms and pharmaceutical companies, but in the end they took the offer from DW Healthcare Partners, a private equity firm in Utah with an established track record of bringing companies like Z-Medica to a larger scale. From the beginning Bart and Frank had a good feeling about the DW Healthcare team, which agreed to Bart and Frank's two nonnegotiable requirements: that the headquarters of Z-Medica, after the purchase, remain in Connecticut and that the company retain every single one of its employees. Bart, of course, took the lead in the negotiations. During the prolonged discussions, Frank showed virtually no interest in the details or even the terms of a deal. At one point Bart and Frank were in a meeting in which $30 million was on the line. Before the meeting Frank had said to Bart, "If we can't work it out in about fifteen minutes, I will have to leave. I am sure you can work it out."

"Really?" Bart had said, surprised—but also not surprised at all.

Indeed, fifteen minutes into the meeting, Frank got up and left.

The deal was struck in the summer of 2012. The terms of the sale were such that Bart and Frank would get two payments each, one at the close of the deal in the fall of 2012 and another, even larger check in four years, after, it was presumed, DW Partners had grown Z-Medica significantly. In one of their last major company decisions, in April 2012, Bart and Frank donated $800,000 worth of QuikClot to hospitals and refugee camps in Syria.

Now, in the Bank of America parking lot, after depositing his check and after he stopped howling and slamming the steering wheel so much that his fists hurt, Bart's first call was to Frank.

"Did you get your check too?" Bart said.

"Yes I did," Frank said. Bart could almost feel Frank smiling on the other end of the phone, all the way in West Hartford.

Bart knew, but did not begrudge the fact, that Frank's payment was significantly larger. After all, Frank was the inventor. None of it could have occurred without Frank. But then again, none of it could have occurred without Bart either.

"We did good, Frank," Bart said.

"We did," Frank said.

"Real good."

"Couldn't have done it without you," Frank said.

"No, you couldn't have!" Bart said. "That's for damn sure."

There was a pause in the conversation for a moment. Neither of them knew what to say next.

Then Bart said, "That'll do, Frank. That'll do."

Frank laughed.

"Yeah, that'll do," Frank said.

Often Bart's cultural references were lost on Frank—there was that crucial six-year difference in their ages—but here Frank knew exactly what Bart was alluding to. Bart was quoting the movie *Babe*, which Frank had watched with his grandkids. In the movie, an eccentric Australian farmer enters his pig, Babe, into a sheepherding competition. After Babe wins the grand prize, the farmer looks down at his pig and says tenderly, "That'll do, pig. That'll do." Frank and Bart both knew that what they had pulled off was as improbable as a pig winning a sheepherding competition.

The check cleared in one business day, on Monday, just like every other check Bart had deposited in his life. Bart had assumed that somehow it would take longer. There was now an additional $12 million in his bank account, with much more on the way. But it was only when Bart saw the numbers on the bank statement, looking very staid and official and somehow permanent in black ink, that the reality of what had occurred set in. It didn't quite seem possible, or even fathomable, that not much more than a decade ago he was turned down for a hundred jobs in a row and Frank struggled to pay his heating bills.

With the money, Bart soon bought a beachfront house in Old Saybrook. The Connecticut shore is notoriously craggy, but Bart found a property located on a small bluff along an unusually long and half-mile-wide stretch of beach. The house had commanding views of Long Island Sound all the way to the North Fork of Long Island. It was twenty-five miles away from Connecticut College, where he had begun his career, and only forty miles away, across the sound, from Southampton College, where he'd had his last job before setting out to be an entrepreneur. It was also two blocks from the cottage in which he had spent summers as a kid, where his father had bullied him for much of his youth. In buying a far nicer house than his parents had, Bart hoped that he could reclaim or rewrite his family narrative and start again.

He also bought a snazzy condo in Jupiter, Florida, on the water. And, after drinking too much champagne at a boat show in Fort Lauderdale, he had a lapse in judgment, wrote a check for $1 million, and bought a yacht. The boat was gorgeous and sleek, made by a prestigious manufacturer, a forty-two-foot center console craft with four outboard motors. But, as Bart soon found out, the yacht was disastrously engineered. "I will never drink too much at a boat show again," he joked to Frank. In retirement—actually semiretirement, because managing his investments soon became a part-time job—Bart became the ultimate Connecticut-to-Florida snowbird. He spends December to June in Florida and July to Thanksgiving in Connecticut. These days he drives up and down the East Coast in the RV and has developed an encyclopedic knowledge of the best local restaurants along the way, sometimes detouring for hours just to get the best crab cake in Baltimore, the best grits and sausage in eastern North Carolina, the best oysters in Connecticut, or the best blueberry pancakes in Maine. Joe Dacorta, who remains a friend, recalled going out for breakfast with Bart in Virginia. Asked for his order, Bart told the waiter, "We'll have the left side of the menu." Often he leaves a hundred-dollar tip.

He sold the elegant but malfunctioning yacht a few years later, at a loss. Realizing he couldn't rid himself of the harassing ghost of his father, he sold the Old Saybrook house too. He even got rid of the Jupiter condo. Most of the people in the development were eighty or ninety years old, and the incessant sound of the bridges opening on the Intracoastal Waterway kept him up at night. Instead he bought a handsome but simpler home twenty minutes away in Niantic, not far from the Pfizer ghetto he had lived in ten years previously. The house is on the Niantic River, which is really an estuary, and Bart surveys its tidal waters each morning as he has coffee. In Florida he bought a well-appointed but also not extravagant house in a gated community in Palm Beach Gardens, just a block away from where he had lived with Linda a decade before.

Bart never remarried. He lives alone, although he has plenty of regular guests, including many old friends. He still dates occasionally but is not in a committed relationship. In his seventies Bart has gone about the hard work of his emotional recovery, recognizing his history of shortcomings with his family. He is arriving at a sense of peace and contentment about the unquiet path that he has traveled, filled as it was with difficulties and deep loss but also profound triumph. He still suffers from clinical depression. "I think I had depression from the moment I was born," he says. "I think my father had it." He is successfully in therapy, which has been reduced over time from three sessions a week to one, with an excellent counselor. His goal is to continue to treat and manage his depression and, more than anything, to find emotional stability in his relationship with his daughter. He realizes that it was his own failings that led to their separation after her adolescent years when Bart was suffering his breakdown. These days the true center of his life is Sarah. Like him, she became a rower in college, at College of the Holy Cross in Massachusetts. She lives in Montreal, but she and Bart are in touch regularly. His greatest hope is that they will come to understand each other fully before he dies.

Quietly, Bart has given money away to Connecticut high school crew programs and beach conservation organizations. In 2015, after hearing of a devastating earthquake in Nepal through a Nepalese doctor who had worked at Z-Medica, Bart organized a fundraiser and campaign to send nine thousand sheets of corrugated galvanized steel to that country to help provide temporary shelter and roofs in aid of the 100,000 people who were injured in the event. He has also given significant money to Yale New Haven Hospital, where he underwent heart bypass surgery in 2016, when it was discovered after tests that he had six blocked arteries. The surgery went well and only a few months afterward Bart felt that he had been granted an entirely new lease on life. A few years ago, Bart loaned $4 million to a friend from his days in the Hamptons, a once-near-billionaire who had gone bankrupt.

In 2020, after having grown multiple times over during an eight-year period, Z-Medica was sold to Teleflex, a large medical device company based in Pennsylvania, for $500 million. One of the reasons for the size of the sale was that Combat Gauze had finally begun to penetrate the hospital market and was now being used in the growing number of surgeries for the aging population. By this point Bart and Frank had been paid out completely, and they personally did not profit from the sale. Still, they took a great deal of satisfaction from the news. Frank in particular found it mind-boggling that the results of his experiment in the basement of his West Hartford home thirty-five years earlier had been sold for half a billion dollars.

While Z-Medica thrived, its old competitor and nemesis, Hem-Con, declared bankruptcy and was sold at the fire-sale price of $3 million in 2013. HemCon's sales had almost completely evaporated after the introduction of Combat Gauze in 2008, and in 2010 the company lost a $29.4 million lawsuit for patent infringement.

A company called Marine Polymer, which had entered its own product in the original Alam trial, successfully sued HemCon for stealing its idea of using chitosan as a blood clotting agent. In 2012 HemCon canceled all existing stocks, leaving behind a trail of apoplectic investors. Jody Stahancyk, a Portland attorney who bought nearly 30 percent of the first round of HemCon shares, wrote to the HemCon board of directors, "You each deserve a special place in hell for not facing the shareholders who invested in you....When the [HemCon] patent died, each of you Board Members should have signed the letter and made personal calls to shareholders. Your failure to be personally accountable speaks volumes of each of your lack of personal character."

Combat Gauze is now a ubiquitous product. Pop star Taylor Swift made international news when she said in 2019, "I carry QuikClot army grade bandage dressing, which is for gunshot or stab wounds." Swift explained that she was afraid of violence at her concerts. "After the Manchester Arena bombing and the Vegas concert shooting, I was completely terrified to go on tour...because I didn't know how we were going to keep three million fans safe over seven months," she said. Combat Gauze is standard in many police departments, including in New York and Chicago. It was used by first responders at the Boston Marathon bombing, the Parkland school shooting in Florida, and the Mandalay Bay hotel shootings in Las Vegas. Before the Las Vegas shootings, every vehicle of that city's metropolitan police department had been issued a trauma kit including Combat Gauze. In a subsequently published police report about the Mandalay Bay shooting, which occurred in 2018, a Sergeant Kennedy noted that Detective William Ghilarducci "applied quick clot [sic] gauze to some of the bullet wounds on [redacted name] and [redacted name]" because one of the people shot "was bleeding profusely as she was hit in multiple spots." Ghilarducci, Kennedy noted, had significant experience and military training relevant to such situations. During transport to the hospital, Ghilarducci continued to treat and calm one of the wounded people, who appeared to be going into shock from blood loss. Both of the wounded civilians Ghilarducci assisted survived and made full recoveries. That same year, in New York City, a two-year-old girl's life was saved by Combat Gauze when her body was sliced open by a falling glass shower door. Bart and Frank have Google news alerts set up for the terms "QuikClot" and "Combat Gauze," and every few months or so, almost without fail, a story like this pops up. A man on Cape Cod is saved after a shark attack; a woman in Wyoming is saved after being cut by a lawn mower blade; a wounded dog is saved by its owner; a criminal is saved after having been shot by a police officer; a police officer, shot by a criminal, is saved by a fellow officer. These stories, which Bart reads on his computer while sitting on his patio in Florida or poolside in Connecticut, make him realize anew that all his struggles and troubles, even his breakdown, were worth it. Frank reads them in West Hartford and smiles and says a prayer of gratitude for what he and Bart were able to accomplish together.

As Bart looks back on his life—he is seventy-four now, the same age as his father when he died—he can see that it was not an uninteresting one. Bart has won most of his battles, even if the price has been considerable. He has learned that forgiveness can bring peace. He now realizes that his father, who degraded him so, suffered from his own untreated clinical depression and war trauma, and he has forgiven his father for how he behaved. His father's lacerating voice, which plagued him for decades, has diminished to a whisper. At this point much of the pain has faded away, and the humor and absurdity of his misadventures, rather than the missteps, are what he recalls. Now he realizes that until he met Frank at Paradise Pizza in 1999, everything in his life—except for his daughter—was prologue. If it weren't for Frank and Sarah, he might well be a bouncer somewhere, or a truck driver, or living out of hotels. He might be dead. Quiet, inimitable Frank changed everything.

For his part, Frank, despite his newfound wealth, has never really changed. In his late seventies, he still goes into the offices of On-Site, although now his visits are infrequent. He still lives in the same modest house where he discovered zeolite. Mostly he spends time with Nancy and his children and grandchildren, as well as at the local Catholic Church he attends weekly. Of course, he is now fabulously wealthy, his net worth comparable to the endowment of a small college. He still seems slightly shocked at this development, often wearing a look of surprise and mild amusement at where he, a small-town kid from Dillon, South Carolina, has ended up. Whenever someone brings up his success, he chuckles awkwardly and typically shifts the conversation.

He also likes to give his money away, but in bigger amounts than Bart. He has given significant sums to his alma mater, the University of Hartford, to the local nature center, to the parks and recreation department of his hometown in South Carolina, and to the Boy Scouts. He made one of his biggest donations through his parish in West Hartford. Frank's priest there is originally from Uganda and had many times shared with Frank the dire needs of youth in his native country. Having fond memories of summer camp in South Carolina, Frank, with Nancy, financed the building of an attractive, air-conditioned fifteen-room hotel in the city of Soroti in eastern Uganda, the proceeds of which would support a youth summer camp. The Hursey Resort in Soroti opened in 2016. It turned out there was extraordinary karma in the donation. A year after the hotel was built, Nancy was in dire need of a kidney transplant.

One of the priest's parishioners, newly moved to Connecticut, was a match and donated her kidney to Nancy in a procedure at the University of Massachusetts Memorial Medical Center.

Frank has also become a real estate tycoon of sorts and the owner of a limousine company. In 2004, somewhat impulsively, for Frank at least, he bought an oceanfront colonial house in the town of Dennis on Cape Cod. But Frank really bought the house for Nancy, who loved being near the ocean and found it good for her health. Two houses down from the beachfront house was a nondescript thirty-three-bed seasonal hotel overlooking Nantucket Sound. The owner sold the hotel in 2007. The building was converted into time-shares that proved largely unsuccessful, and the building deteriorated. In 2018 Frank and his son-in-law, an accomplished real estate developer, purchased the property with the idea of converting it back to a hotel but on a grander scale. Frank was the lead investor, but there were ten others. A good portion of the money invested was loaned by Bart. The group led a $9 million renovation that ballooned to a cost of $20 million. The project involved gutting every room to the studs and building an additional two-story building with a restaurant and retractable roof. The newly opened Pelham House Resort opened in the summer of 2020, the first summer of the pandemic, and offered open-air rooftop dining. It was overrun by demand. Next Frank bought a nearby motel where the Pelham House hotel workers could stay. Then he bought a house on six acres that his grandson operates as an Airbnb and a farm that provides produce for the Pelham. Then, with cash continuing to flow in at Pelham House, Frank bought a twenty-seven-room hotel in the downtown area of West Dennis. Finally, in the spring of 2022, Frank's group bought a fourth hotel in the area. Frank's consortium, now a mini empire, has been written up enthusiastically by the *Boston Globe* and *Condé*

Nast Traveler. Frank and Nancy also personally maintain an ocean-side home in his native South Carolina. Frank remains fit and trim, and with his full head of salt-and-pepper hair, he looks quite a bit younger than his age. Now he wears blazers more frequently than he used to, and he has taken on a professorial, even vaguely aristocratic look. But he is as modest and as self-effacing as ever.

In the fall of 2021, with a massive donation from Frank and Nancy, the University of Hartford, Frank's alma mater from ten years of night school, opened the newly constructed Francis X. and Nancy Hursey Center for Advanced Engineering and Health Professions, a state-of-the-art sixty-thousand-square-foot building in the center of campus. As Frank likes to say, the school is a perfect combination of their interests and careers: Frank's as an engineer and Nancy's as a nurse. The facility is home to laboratories and classrooms, including a "health simulation" suite, a space that mimics a hospital with four treatment rooms in which students simulate their future work in assessing, diagnosing, and treating patients in the form of lifelike robots. The engineering quarters of the facility include work spaces for robotics, 3D printing, and cybersecurity labs.

The entire Hursey family attended the grand opening on an overcast day in September 2021. Frank and Nancy's three children and all their grandchildren were given a tour of the facility. The event was gleefully organized by senior officials from the university, and in attendance were CEOs and executives from the blue-chip Hartford-area corporations that had also donated to the project, including Pratt & Whitney (where Frank worked as an engineer's aide when he first came to Hartford), Hartford Hospital (where he worked in the respiratory department), the Hartford Steam Boiler Inspection and Insurance Company, and Stanley Black & Decker. It was the royalty of Hartford industry and technology, and over the course of the ceremony, Frank was feted by all of them.

He was called to the podium by the provost. He was wearing a gold medal, the university's highest alumni award, which he had been awarded previously. Nancy sat in a wheelchair by his side. Frank expressed his appreciation to the University of Hartford for sticking by him in the decade it took for him to get his degree, and he thanked one engineering professor in particular who had given him a mediocre grade but also taken him aside and said that he had unusual talent and vision and might one day make a contribution to the field. Frank told the crowd that he had created an oxygen and nitrogen gas company, and then, with a partner, built another company that developed a blood clotting agent. "Then we had a fight with the army," Frank said. "But we won. In the end, it all worked out pretty well." He chuckled. After speaking for only about five minutes, he stopped abruptly, saying, "Well, that's about all I got." The audience seemed simultaneously charmed and slightly confused by the brevity of the speech. They clearly wanted to know more, but Frank had made it clear that was all he wanted to say. Afterward, university administrators triumphantly conducted tours for guests and local reporters. Frank participated for a little while but soon drifted away to a corner of the lab, where he sat with Nancy and played with the youngest of his grandchildren.

Privately, however, far away from an audience, Frank says there is much he would still like to achieve scientifically, and if he were younger, he would undertake it. He believes, for example, that there is still much untapped potential in zeolite. He has used ground-up zeolite as a treatment for an extended family member's bedsores and was struck by how quickly they healed. Unglamorous bedsores, which are a form of ulcer, are a major health problem among the bedbound elderly, and they can quickly turn into serious infections, even leading to death. To Frank's knowledge no one has explored zeolite as a treatment. "It could be a game changer,"

Frank says. He also believes that the pressure swing technology he developed in his oxygen and nitrogen machines can be made much more efficient. But, he says, getting all the calibrations exactly right would take years. "If I was twenty, that's what I would do," he says. "I would spend five years refining the capabilities of pressure swing technology."

But other than the event at the University of Hartford, the only formal recognition that Frank has ever received from the scientific community is his brief mention by *Scientific American* in 2003, when he was named as one of the top fifty "research leaders of the year" for the original formulation of QuikClot. To date, not a single journal article has been written about him or his work. His name is never mentioned in the scientific papers on the hemostatic properties of zeolite. In the field of medicine, he is completely unknown. The man who saw things that no one else could see—and who did it twice, once each for zeolite *and* kaolin—is himself invisible. There are scientists who have won the Nobel Prize for less. Frank changed the paradigm; he not only halted bleeding, he also took bleeding control largely out of the hands of doctors—with their vials of Factor Seven—and put it into the hands of police officers, EMTs, adventurers, soldiers, hikers, and moms and dads. Bart believes Frank's unique genius is making complex things simple. He sees Frank as the "Ringo Starr of inventors": like the Beatles' drummer, he is able to distill things down to a level of disarming and brilliant simplicity. Frank and Bart are also intensely proud that their work in creating QuikClot was essentially self-funded: in stark contrast to the HemCon and fibrin bandages, QuikClot received only minimal government support. But Frank, of course, holds no animosity about his lack of acclaim. The satisfaction of saving lives, and his fortune, are enough.

Bart and Frank never quite know what to say when they are

confronted, as they are quite regularly, with the story of a person whose life was saved by QuikClot. Bart was doing business at the bank in Old Saybrook when the assistant manager told him that QuikClot kept him alive in Iraq. Bart's mind usually flashes to the Hebrew saying, "Save one life, and you save the entire world." But Frank and Bart are sure to take no direct credit for anyone's survival. There are too many factors and causes behind any one soldier's or victim's predicament. All that Frank and Bart acknowledge is that they stayed the course and brought the product to the people who needed it.

But one story of survival hit Bart hard when he read about it in a New Jersey newspaper. It seemed to bring home everything that had occurred in his life, and what he accomplished since he met Frank, in a way that nothing had before. Nearly twenty years after Jamie Smith's death in Mogadishu, on January 30, 2010, a twenty-six-year-old policeman drove to the Fairfield, New Jersey, station to report for his 7:00 p.m. shift. Fairfield, a suburb of Newark, is twenty miles east of the town where Jamie Smith grew up. It was a bitter, dark night, 5 degrees outside. The officer, Gerald Veneziano, still wearing street clothes, was driving a silver Volkswagen Passat. A black Dodge had been tailgating him recklessly for some miles and flashing its headlights. Veneziano pulled into a parking lot two blocks from the police station. The driver of the Dodge sidled up next to Veneziano's car. Veneziano rolled down his window and identified himself as a policeman. Without a word the other driver, who would later be identified as Preye Roberts, pulled out a gun and shot Veneziano in the face. Then Roberts got out of his car, shot Veneziano seven more times, and drove away. When it was all over, Veneziano lay in the parking lot with a shattered jaw, a broken femur, two collapsed lungs, and three bullets in his left leg. He was the first officer in the seventy-three-year history of the town to be shot. Someone in the vicinity heard the shots, and, believing them to be fireworks, called in a noise complaint to the police station. Bleeding voluminously from multiple bullet entrance and exit wounds all over his body, Veneziano somehow crawled to the roadway thirty yards away. He lay by the road as two cars slowed down but didn't stop. Veneziano was certain he was going to die. Weirdly, it was a peaceful, almost light feeling, an ebbing away of cares and sensation. Finally a third driver, an eighteen-year-old man driving home from the gym, stopped and called 911. Police officers arrived in minutes, sank to their knees, and began bandaging Veneziano's jaw. Veneziano said, "Tell my parents I love them. Tell my girlfriend I'm sorry."

"Tell them yourself," an officer said.

"Work on my leg, not my jaw," he told an officer. Veneziano could feel the blood pouring out of his thigh. He had been an EMT before he joined the police and knew that he had been hit in the femoral artery and that the injury would be fatal if left untreated. An officer opened a first-aid kit, pulled out Combat Gauze, and applied it to the wound. Half an hour later, Veneziano was in the hospital in Newark, where he was put into a medically induced coma. He was operated on for twelve hours and then spent two weeks in the intensive care unit and two and a half months in a rehabilitation hospital.

Gerald Veneziano is thirty-seven now. He has extensive nerve damage, a rod in his femur, and a damaged jaw. He returned to the police force, but his anxiety forced him to leave after four years. He married the sister of the man who found him in the roadway and is now a foreman at a concrete plant and has two children.

Two young men, both from northern New Jersey, both shot in the femoral artery. One lived, one died. The only difference was that Veneziano was treated with something that Bart Gullong and Frank

Hursey had brought into the world eight years after Jamie Smith died. Had they gotten there earlier, Smith could have lived.

These days Bart spends a lot of time alone, thinking about the past. He is pensive but content. He is acutely grateful for the substantial contributions of the people "who got it," particularly the tireless employees of Z-Medica. In Connecticut he spends hours by the pool, sometimes spotting bald eagles in the trees. For some reason his mind often wanders to one particular afternoon in high school. It was during the time at Tabor when he was deemed too uncoordinated and ungraceful to play basketball or football and backed into the crew team. One afternoon Bart and the team were rowing out on the open water well beyond the safety of the harbor of Buzzards Bay—a challenging proposition on a good day, but a daunting, even dangerous one if the winds were high. As the winds picked up, the waves battered the boat, and the icy water spilled into the shell. A gale descended from the sky and blew the boat far out into the bay. Suddenly the boat was two miles from shore. Bart—new to rowing but not to seamanship—took over from the panicked coxswain and became the crew's navigator. He yelled at the squad to drive the boat diagonally into the waves—so as to avoid the full head-on force of the water—and to focus together on their technique, sit up, and drive their legs. For the longest minute it seemed that the shell would either sink or be thrown helplessly farther out to sea. But finally, inch by inch and then foot by foot, they gained control of the boat. Eventually they made their way out of the rip and into calmer water. By the time they arrived at the dock, Bart crumpled into himself with exhaustion. At the same time, he had never felt more exhilarated.

He had given everything he had, until there was nothing left to give.

Author's Note and Acknowledgments

This book is not a history of the Z-Medica and On-Site Gas Systems companies but rather focuses primarily on the work of Bart Gullong and Frank Hursey. In the interests of focusing the narrative, the contributions of many worthy employees have not been described, but their collective work was of course instrumental in QuikClot's success. At times names have been changed in the interests of privacy.

My deepest gratitude is to my wife and son. My wife, Laura, showed extraordinary forbearance and loyalty to this project, as well as much sage advice and guidance. I literally could not have done it without her. My son, Louis, whose own writing shows so much promise, has been wonderfully supportive. My brothers, Tom and John, as always, have assisted in ways large and small. I very much wish that my late parents, Sheila and Bill—each of them forged by experiences in combat or wartime—could read this account.

I would like to thank my colleagues at Wesleyan and Yale who read draft material and generally offered goodwill. These include Michael Rowe, Andrew Curran, Sean McCann, Tushar Irani, Michael Roth, and Kari Weil. I would also like to thank doctors Ian Roberts, Hasan Alam, and Stephan Mayer for their expert consultation and also for their reading of the manuscript. Other doctors and experts on bleeding who I interviewed and graciously offered their expertise were Vernoica Yank, Louis Aledort, Nigel Key, Jawed Fareed, Timothy Hodgetts, and Yulia Lin. Also the veterans Ryan Kules and Seth Secrease bravely shared their combat experiences, and Gerald Veneziano shared his story as a New Jersey police officer.

I would like to deeply thank fellow writers Jeff Hobbs and Robert Kolker for early and much valued support of the project. I am in particular debt to Robert Little. He shared with remarkable generosity his knowledge of the larger story, as well as background material. I also relied on his first-class reporting in the *Baltimore Sun*.

I was the beneficiary of timely research support, funded by Wesleyan, and the research assistance of the Wesleyan undergraduates or now alumni: Peter Dunphy, Sofia Khu, Ben Owen, and Emma Dhanda. Ben and Sofia did many months of superb work on this project, and Sofia additionally wrote draft material.

I would like to thank my longtime wonderful agent, and friend, Dan Conaway. Also, I am grateful to Sean Daily of Hotchkiss Daily and Associates for his work, as well as Timothy and Trevor White, and Joey and Abigail Hartstone of Star Thrower Entertainment.

The team at Grand Central Publishing—Colin Dickerman, Rachael Kelly, and Jen McArdle—have been unfailingly responsive, helpful, and extremely diligent. Colin is simply the best editor I have ever worked with.

I appreciate the contributions of the following who assisted in various ways: Sanh Phan, Dennis White, Christine Tappe, Jane Marsh, Tyler Garzo, and Michael Gross of the Authors Guild. I would like to thank the family members of the Hursey and Gullong families, in particular Nancy and Sarah. Finally, I would like to honor and acknowledge the memories of Jessica Perkins and Thomas "Tommy" Eagles.

Of course my deepest appreciation goes to Josepha Dacorta, Timothy Coakley, Frank Hursey, and Bart Gullong for opening the full extent of their experiences and the deepest recesses of their souls to me. Bart Gullong has been exceptionally honest and forthcoming, and his unstinting humor and dedication have been much valued over the many years of the birthing of this account. I will forever be grateful to all four of them.

Endnotes

PRELUDE: MOGADISHU, 1993

"A protracted conflict between Aidid and his rivals": "Somalia Faces the Future: Human Rights in a Fragmented Society." *Human Rights Watch* 7, no. 2, April 1995. https://www.hrw.org/reports/1995/somalia/

"The military strategists—both Americans and advisers from NATO forces—believed that the mission would be accomplished within ninety minutes": "Ambush in Mogadishu," synopsis, *Frontline*, PBS.org, Sept. 29, 1998. https://www.pbs.org/wgbh/pages/frontline/shows/ambush/etc/synopsis.html

"little more than a quick 'snatch-and-grab' operation": Mark Bowden, "The Legacy of Black Hawk Down." *Smithsonian Magazine,* January 2019.

"fell ninety feet to the ground": Alisa Adams, "Honoring Army Veteran Todd Blackburn, 25th Anniversary of Battle of Mogadishu." *VA News*, Oct. 13, 2018. https://news.va.gov/52992/todd-blackburn-25th-anniversary-battle-of-mogadishu/

"The two pilots were killed instantly": Captain Frank K. Butler, "Tactical Management of Urban Warfare Casualties in Special Operations." *Military Medicine* 165, supplement 1, 2000. https://watermark.silverchair.com/milmed-165-suppl_1-1

"shots to the pelvis and abdomen": "The Battle of Mogadishu," U.S. Army Airborne & Special Operations Museum website. https://www.asomf.org/the-battle-of-mogadishu/

"Furthermore, shooting one into the sky": Mark Bowden, *Black Hawk Down: A Story of Modern War* (New York: Penguin Books, 2000), 88.

"afraid to die": Ibid., 109–110.

"the longest sustained conflict in which the American military had been engaged since Vietnam": R. L. Mabry, J. B. Holcomb, A. M. Baker, C. C. Cloonan, J. M. Uhorchak, D. E. Perkins, A. J. Canfield, and J. H. Hagmann, "United States Army Rangers in Somalia: An Analysis of Combat Casualties on an Urban Battlefield." *Journal of Trauma* 49, no. 3, 2000.

ENDNOTES

"In the end, he was given only ten seconds' notice that casualties were inbound": John B. Holcomb, M.D., guest, "Blood Product Resuscitation," May 4, 2015, in *Behind the Knife* podcast, 77 min. https://behindtheknife.org/podcast/7-john-b-holcomb-m-d-ut-houston-blood-product-resuscitation/

"'accidents' are really predictable": "Holcomb, John B., M.D., FACS" (faculty profile), the University of Alabama at Birmingham. https://www.uab.edu/medicine/surgery/trauma/faculty/holcomb

"Holcomb grew up in the 1960s and 1970s in Fort Smith, Arkansas": Liz Caldwell, "'Distinguished Alumnus' Honored by College of Medicine." *UAMS News*, Sept. 4, 2013. https://news.uams.edu/2013/09/04/distinguished-alumnus-honored-by-college-of-medicine/

"lowest cost of living in the United States": City Wire staff, "Kiplinger: Fort Smith least expensive city in the U.S." *Talk Business & Politics*, August 2, 2010. https://talkbusiness.net/2010/08/kiplinger-fort-smith-least-expensive-city-in-u-s/

"manufacturing and processing centers for Planters peanut": Aric Mitchell, "Planters Peanuts Celebrates 35 Years in Fort Smith, Donates Food." *Talk Business & Politics*, May 25, 2011. https://talkbusiness.net/2011/05/planters-peanuts-celebrates-35-years-in-fort-smith-donates-food/

"He chose the army because his father had been an army officer": John B. Holcomb, MD, FACS, "Special Operations Surgeon Uses Lessons Learned in Somalia to Revolutionize Combat Casualty Care in the Global War on Terrorism" and "Innovations in Hemorrhage Control and Transfusion Paradigms Redefining Trauma Combat Casualty Care Guidelines," Parts 1 and 2, *WarDocs—The Military Medicine Podcast*, April 11 and 16, 2022. https://wardocspodcast.podbean.com

"After receiving his medical degree from the University of Arkansas in 1985": John Bradley Holcomb CV. https://docplayer.net/15548393-John-bradley-holcomb-m-d-f-a-c-s.html

"'a very capable hospital'": John B. Holcomb, "Capital Preservation: Preparing for Urban Operations in the 21st Century" (presentation, RAND Arroyo-TRADOC-MCWL-OSD Urban Operations Conference, March 22–23, 2000).

"The wounded and the dying arrived in two waves": Ibid.

"Out of the two hundred combatants in the conflict, 112 were injured and seventy were hospitalized": Ibid.

"The first three or four patients Holcomb operated on died": "Blood Product Resuscitation," May 4, 2015, in *Behind the Knife* podcast.

"despite being given forty-six pints of blood": Avram Goldstein, "Hope of Survival Wrapped in a Simple Bandage." *Washington Post*, May 12, 1999.

"elbow deep in a soldier's abdomen": "A Tribute to Medical Task Force 46: Their Story during the Battle of Mogadishu," John M. Uhorchak, the Veterans Site. https://blog.theveteranssite.greatergood.com/uhorchak-tribute/

"operated by flashlight": R. L. Mabry, J. B. Holcomb, A. M. Baker, C. C. Cloonan, J. M. Uhorchak, D. E. Perkins, A. J. Canfield, and J. H. Hagmann, "United States Army Rangers in Somalia: An Analysis of Combat Casualties on an Urban Battlefield." *Journal of Trauma* 49, no. 3, 2000.

"'bled to death in my hands'": Margo Shideler, Finding Meaning and Leading

Through Tragedy, *Encircle*, Centenary College Alumni Magazine, Spring 2012. https://www.centenary.edu/files/resources/encircle-spring-2012.pdf

"Holcomb would refer to the entire blood-soaked episode as 'the defining experience of my life'": "Blood Product Resuscitation," May 4, 2015, in *Behind the Knife* podcast.

"'To have those soldiers bleed to death'": Usha Lee McFarling, "New Bandage Creates Instant Blood Clots; Dealing with Blood Loss Hasn't Changed Since Days of Roman Legions." *Lewiston Tribune*, March 3, 1999. https://lmtribune.com/northwest/new-bandage-creates-instant-blood-clots-dealing-with-blood-loss-hasnt-changed-since-days-of/article_acc69ced-92ed-5f43-873b-ec9638b91db3.html

"events in Mogadishu took place during a high-water mark": "Author Mark Bowden Revisits the True Story of 'Black Hawk Down.'" Military.com, May 13, 2019. https://www.military.com/daily-news/2019/05/13/author-mark-bowden-revisits-true-story-black-hawk-down.html

"President Bill Clinton ordered all American soldiers to withdraw": Paul Alexander, "Fallout from Somalia Still Haunts U.S. Policy 20 Years Later." *Stars and Stripes*, October 3, 2013. https://www.stripes.com/news/fallout-from-somalia-still-haunts-us-policy-20-years-later-1.244957

"'The extent of your impotence and weaknesses became very clear'": Mark Danner, "Taking Stock of the Forever War." *New York Times Magazine*, Sept. 11, 2005. https://www.nytimes.com/2005/09/11/magazine/taking-stock-of-the-forever-war.html

"'it turned my career a hundred and eighty degrees'": "Special Operations Surgeon Uses Lessons Learned in Somalia to Revolutionize Combat Casualty Care in the Global War on Terrorism" and "Innovations in Hemorrhage Control and Transfusion Paradigms Redefining Trauma Combat Casualty Care Guidelines," Parts 1 and 2, *WarDocs—The Military Medicine Podcast*.

"'Unfortunately, we are currently surrounding our soldiers with incredible technology'": Holcomb, "Capital Preservation" (presentation).

"'rapid' and 'relevant,' techniques, even if those techniques were 'unproved [sic] but [made] sense'": Ibid.

"'young people who must have good hands'": Ibid.

CHAPTER ONE: THE SIMPLEST IDEA

"surface area of a football field": U.S. Geological Survey, "Mineral Resource of the Month: Zeolites." *EARTH*, Oct. 3, 2014. https://www.earthmagazine.org/article/mineral-resource-month-zeolites/

CHAPTER TWO: ALL BLEEDING STOPS EVENTUALLY

"even controversial treatments were 'amazing'": Robert Little, "Dangerous Remedy." *Baltimore Sun*, Nov. 19, 2006.

"'good for patients'": J. B. Holcomb and D. H. Jenkins, "Get Ready: Whole Blood Is Back and It's Good for Patients." *Transfusion* 58, no. 8, August 2018.

"all while holding down three jobs": "Special Operations Surgeon Uses Lessons Learned in Somalia to Revolutionize Combat Casualty Care in the Global War on Terrorism" and "Innovations in Hemorrhage Control and Transfusion Paradigms Redefining Trauma Combat Casualty Care Guidelines," Parts 1 and 2, *WarDocs—The Military Medicine Podcast.*

"'Wars always cause improvements in trauma care'": "Docs Test 'Suspended Animation' as Potential Battlefield Treatment," A. Chris Gajilan, CNN.com, Nov. 13, 2006. http://www.cnn.com/2006/HEALTH/11/10/golden.hour/

"'Medicine is the only victor in war'": Michael S. Baker, MC USN (Ret.), "Casualties of the Global War on Terror and Their Future Impact on Health Care and Society: A Looming Public Health Crisis." *Military Medicine* 179, no. 4, April 2014.

"the first significant use of anesthesia": Laura Cutter and Tim Clarke Jr., "Anesthesia Advances During the Civil War." *Military Medicine* 179, no. 12, December 2014.

"the regular practice of blood transfusions": J. P Aymard and P. Renaudier, "Blood Transfusion during World War I (1914–1918)." *History of Medical Sciences* 50, no. 3, July 2016.

"The field of chemotherapy was born": S. L. Smith, "War! What Is It Good For? Mustard Gas Medicine." *Canadian Medical Association Journal* 189, no. 8, Feb. 27, 2017.

"World War II saw the expanded use of antibiotics, specifically penicillin": R. Quinn, "Rethinking Antibiotic Research and Development: World War II and the Penicillin Collaborative." *American Journal of Public Health* 103, no. 3, March 2013.

"Doctors in the Vietnam War pioneered the use of frozen blood products": C. R. Valeri, C. E. Brodine, and G. E. Moss, "Use of Frozen Blood in Vietnam." *Bibliotheca Haematologica* 29,1968.

"extraordinary advances in burn care": B. S. Atiyeh, S. W. Gunn, and S. N. Hayek, "Military and Civilian Burn Injuries during Armed Conflicts." *Annals of Burns and Fire Disasters* 20, no. 4, Dec. 31, 2007.

"an 'amiable juice'": Rose George, *Nine Pints: A Journey through the Money, Medicine and Mysteries of Blood* (New York: Henry Holt, 2018), 6.

"the Bible mentions blood more than four hundred times": "Blood," King James Bible Dictionary. https://kingjamesbibledictionary.com/Dictionary/blood

"is about sixty thousand miles long": George, *Nine Pints*, 6.

"'trauma is the least scientific of all major medical disciplines'": D. Demetriades, MD, PhD, FACS, "Trauma: From Inception to Date—Successes, Trials, Errors and Challenges" (presentation, WVU School of Medicine Department of Surgery, 2016). https://www.youtube.com/watch?v=PKwatnID-Ws

"'to adopt new flashy practices without any scientific evidence'": Ibid.

"fourth leading cause of death in the world": C. D. Mathers, D. Joncar, *Updated Projections of Global Mortality and Burden of Disease, 2002–2030: Data Sources, Methods and Results. PLoS Med* 3, no. 11, Nov. 2006: e442.

"fifty thousand Americans a year bleed to death": Avram Goldstein, "Hope of Survival Wrapped in a Simple Bandage." *Washington Post*, May 12, 1999.

"leading cause of death for Americans under the age of forty-five": E. R. Donley and J. W. Loyd, "Hemorrhage Control." [Updated 2022 Jul 19]. In: StatPearls [Internet]. Treasure Island (FL): StatPearls Publishing; 2022 Jan. https://www.ncbi.nlm.nih.gov/books/NBK535393/

"The ISR had begun modestly in 1943 as a branch of Halloran General Hospital on Staten Island": "USAISR History," United States Army Institute of Surgical Research. https://usaisr.health.mil/index.cfm/about/history

"For example, some articles by contributors, including those coauthored by Holcomb, were received and accepted within a day or two": J. B. Holcomb, "Use of Recombinant Activated Factor VII to Treat the Acquired Coagulopathy of Trauma." *Journal of Trauma* 28, no. 6, June 2005: 1298–303; P. R. Cordts, L. A. Brosch, J. B. Holcomb, "Now and Then: Combat Casualty Care Policies for Operation Iraqi Freedom and Operation Enduring Freedom Compared with Those of Vietnam," *Journal of Trauma* 64, no. (2 Suppl), Feb. 2008: S14–20.

"'Command is everything'": "Stopping the Bleed: How Army Surgeons Brought Tourniquets Back into the Medical Mainstream," United States Army Institute of Surgical Research. Feb. 5, 2008. https://www.ccems.com/wp-content/uploads/2021/09/US-Army-Institute-of-Surgical-Research-Tourniquets.pdf

"'a colonel and his memo can do almost anything'": Ibid.

"'lethal triad'": Nicola Credland, "Managing the Trauma Patient Presenting with the Lethal Triad." *International Journal of Orthopaedic and Trauma Nursing* 20, Feb. 2016: 45–53.

"a hundred thousand Americans die from clots": "Impact of Blood Clots on the United States," Centers for Disease Control and Prevention. www.cdc.gov/ncbddd/dvt/infographic-impact.html

"The fibrinogen and thrombin were extracted from the milk of genetically altered pigs": Avram Goldstein, "Hope of Survival Wrapped in a Simple Bandage." *Washington Post*, May 12, 1999.

"fibrin glue, fibrin sheet foam, and fibrin powder—materials that were mass-produced from plasma": D. A. Hickman, C. L. Pawlowski, U. D. S. Sekhon, J. Marks, and A. S. Gupta, "Biomaterials and Advanced Technologies for Hemostatic Management of Bleeding." *Advanced Materials*, 30, no. 4., Jan. 2018.

"it contorts itself into a fine, interlacing mesh": I. S. Bayer, "Advances in Fibrin-Based Materials in Wound Repair: A Review." *Molecules* 27, no. 14, 2022.

"'This is really the first significant advance in emergency treatment'": David Dishneau, "Bandage That Stops Bleeding Developed." *Los Angeles Times*, Nov. 8, 1998.

"'This fibrin bandage is the single most important advance in technology for the military'": Avram Goldstein, "Hope of Survival Wrapped in a Simple Bandage." *Washington Post*, May 12, 1999.

"Holcomb himself said that the bandage was going to transform emergency medicine": Ibid.

"reducing blood loss by between 50 and 85 percent": David Dishneau, "Bandage That Stops Bleeding Developed." *Los Angeles Times*, Nov. 8, 1998.

"The climax of the movie focused on the story of Corporal Jamie Smith":

"Cpl James E. Smith," New Jersey Run for the Fallen, 2023. https://www.njrun forthefallen.org/cpl-james-e-smith.html

"His father had been an army captain in Vietnam": Robert Hanley, "The Somalia Mission: Relatives Recount Dreams of 2 Killed in Somalia." *New York Times*, Oct. 7, 1993.

"As described in *Black Hawk Down*, during the opening salvos of the battle": Bowden, *Black Hawk Down*, 209–214, 237–238, 242.

"The request was denied": Mark Bowden, "Black Hawk Down—an American War Story—Men Trapped, and Commanders in Disarray." *Philadelphia Inquirer*, Feb. 3, 1998. https://archive.seattletimes.com/archive/?date=19980203&slug=2732303

"'When fielded in final form'": J. Holcomb, M. MacPhee, S. Hetz, R. Harris, A. Pusateri, and J. Hess, "Efficacy of a Dry Fibrin Sealant Dressing for Hemorrhage Control After Ballistic Injury." *Archives of Surgery* 133, no. 1, 1998.

"was used in combat during the war on terror in Afghanistan": Robert Little, "Stanching Wounds." *Baltimore Sun*, Nov. 20, 2005.

"a member of his staff had told him that for centuries Chinese fishermen": Cinda Becker, "Bloodless Coup Funded by the Army, Oregon Researchers Turn to the Sea to Develop a Revolutionary Bandage That Stanches Heavy Bleeding." *Modern Healthcare*, July 14, 2003.

"'We were just as skeptical as always'": Robert Little, "Stanching Wounds." *Baltimore Sun*, Nov. 20, 2005.

"'It has no known side effects, the performance is amazing in every study we have developed, and the reports from people who actually use the product have been positive'": Ibid.

"The later bankruptcy papers for the HemCon company, filed in 2013, revealed that it had received a total of $76 million in military grants": United States Bankruptcy Court, District of Oregon, In re: Hemcon Technologies, Inc. Debtor. Case No. 12-32652-elp11, February 15, 2013.

CHAPTER FOUR: THE ROWER

"'the biggest thing that has hit Connecticut College since it [went co-ed] has been the appointment of Bart Gullong'": "Cro Bar?" (editorial), *The Pundit* (Connecticut College student newspaper), Oct. 5, 1972.

"'Bart Gullong: Stroke of Genius'": Donald Kane, *The Pundit*, Oct. 1, 1973.

Results chart. H. B. Alam, D. Burris, J. DaCorta, P. Rhee, "Hemorrhage Control in the Battlefield: Role of New Hemostatic Agents." *Military Medicine* 170, no. 1, 2005.

"the second-fastest approval in the administration's history": Nigel Jaquiss, "The Scarlet Letter." *Willamette Week*, July 31, 2012. https://www.wweek.com /portland/article-19504-the-scarlet-letter.html

"It involved buying shrimp shells in bulk from Iceland": Cinda Becker, "Bloodless Coup Funded by the Army, Oregon Researchers Turn to the Sea to Develop a Revolutionary Bandage That Stanches Heavy Bleeding." *Modern Healthcare*, July 14, 2003.

"allocated $4.5 million of procurements": David E. Williams, Sean Kennedy, and Ben Giovine, *2007 Congressional Pig Book Summary* (Washington, D.C.: Citizens against Government Waste, 2007), 4. https://www.cagw.org/sites/default/files/pdf/2007 _Pig_Book.pdf

"boiling the shells in lye or sodium hydroxide to extract the chitosan": "Bandage Made from Shrimp Shells May Save Lives." *VOA News*, May 12, 2003. https://www.voanews.com/a/a-13-a-2003-05-12-8-bandage/393456.html

"The leading medical officer for the Marine Corps, Rear Admiral Robert Hufstader, requested roughly eighty thousand bags": Robert Little, "Stanching Wounds." *Baltimore Sun*, Nov. 20, 2005.

CHAPTER FIVE: THE WOUND-DRESSER

"'Several years have now elapsed since I first became aware that I had accepted, even from my youth'": Rene Descartes, *Discourse on the Method* (United States: Cosimo, Incorporated, 2008).

"with a budget that was at least triple that of any other country's armed forces, on par with the *entire* GNP of some major countries, like Switzerland": Countries with the highest military spending, 2021. Statista Research Department, Aug. 5, 2022. https://www.statista.com/statistics/262742/countries-with-the-highest -military-spending/; Department of Defence, "FY 2003 Defence Budget," February 2002. Michael O'Hanlon and Aaron Moburg-Jones, The Pentagon's Budget. The Brookings Institution, 2002. https://www.brookings.edu/wp-content/uploads/2016/ 06/20021201.pdf; Switzerland GNP 1995–2022, Macrotrends. https://www.macro trends.net/countries/CHE/switzerland/gnp-gross-national-product

"'The game of science is, in principle, without end'": K. R. Popper, *The Logic of Scientific Discovery* (United Kingdom: Routledge, 2002), 32.

"the fealty among marines, which is 'to our Nation, the Corps, and to each other'": *Leading Marines* (MCWP 6-11) (Washington, D.C.: United States Marine Corps, 2014), 1–6. https://www.marines.mil/Portals/1/MCWP%206-11_Part1 .pdf

"'resolved to act upon Land or meant to confine their Services to the Water only'": "From George Washington to Colonel John Cadwalader, 7 December 1776," Founders Online, National Archives. https://founders.archives.gov /documents/Washington/03-07-02-0205 (Original source: Philander D. Chase (ed.), *The Papers of George Washington, Revolutionary War Series*, vol. 7: 21 October 1776–5 January 1777 (Charlottesville: University Press of Virginia, 1997), 268–269.)

"The corps played a crucial role in Washington's raid on Trenton": "Brief History of the United States Marine Corps," Marine Corps University. https://www.usmcu.edu/Research/Marine-Corps-History-Division/Brief-Histories /Brief-History-of-the-United-States-Marine-Corps/

"The corps grew from fifteen thousand regular duty personnel in 1940": "History of the USMCR," staff of the Marine Reserve Centennial Project, Marine Corps Forces Reserve, 2016. https://www.marforres.marines.mil/usmcr100/history/

"'That does away with the Marine Corps'": Victor H. Krulak, *First to Fight: An Inside View of the U.S. Marine Corps* (Naval Institute Press, 1984), 127–8.

"President Harry Truman, who carried a hatred of the marines": "The Marine Corps as the Navy's Police Force." *Marine Corps University.* https://www.usmcu.edu /Research/Marine-Corps-History-Division/Frequently-Requested-Topics/Historical -Documents-Orders-and-Speeches/The-Marine-Corps-as-the-Navys-Police-Force

"the army had nearly three times as many personnel as the marines": Budget FY 2004—Department of Defense—Military," GovInfo. https://www.govinfo.gov /app/details/BUDGET-2004-PER/BUDGET-2004-PER-15-1-5/context

"The distance between the combat zone and the hospital could be 350 miles": Professional Note: Forward Resuscitative Surgery in Operation Iraqi Freedom by Captain H. R. Bohman and Captain Bruce C. Baker, Medical Corps, U.S. Navy, and Captain Rom A. Stevens, Medical Corps, U.S. Naval Reserve February 2004. Vol. 130/2/1,212. U.S. Naval Institute. https://www.usni.org /magazines/proceedings / 2004 / february/professional-note-forward-resuscitative -surgery-operation-iraqi

"Eight of those patients would have died if not for FRSS intervention": L. W. Chambers, P. Rhee, B. C. Baker, J. Perciballi, M. Cubano, M. Compeggie, M. Nace, H. R. Bohman, "Initial Experience of US Marine Corps Forward Resuscitative Surgical System during Operation Iraqi Freedom." *Archives of Surgery* 140, no. 1, Jan. 2005.

CHAPTER SEVEN: "YOU BURN PEOPLE!"

"selected HemCon as the 'hemostatic agent of choice'": Frank K. Butler Jr., MC USN (Ret.), John B. Holcomb, MC USA, Stephen D. Giebner, MD, MPH, Norman E. McSwain, MD, FACS, and James Bagian, MD, "Tactical Combat Casualty Care 2007: Evolving Concepts and Battlefield Experience." *Military Medicine* 172, supplement 1, Nov. 2007.

"The HemCom company received an initial $400,000 grant from the army": Robert Little, "Stanching Wounds." *Baltimore Sun*, Nov. 20, 2005.

"its workforce would reach 120 personnel": Geoff Pursinger, "HemCon Is Moving Out of Tigard." *Tigard Times*, Sept. 4, 2014. https://pamplinmedia.com/ttt /89-news/232458-96860-hemcon-is-moving-out-of-tigard

"'HemCon doesn't work'": Robert Little, "Stanching Wounds," *Baltimore Sun*, Nov. 20, 2005.

"the army from naming HemCon one of its 'Top 10 Greatest Inventions'": Ibid.

"One study showed that it tended to fall out of the wound after an average of forty-nine minutes": Ibid.

"Two studies conducted before the start of the Iraq War found that HemCon functioned no better than gauze": Robert Little, "Untested in Battle." *Baltimore Sun*, March 29, 2009.

"'The Marine Corps does not have any plans to purchase HemCon'": "Update on the Use of Combat Helmets, Vehicle Armor and Body Armor by Ground

Forces in Operation Iraqi Freedom and Operation Enduring Freedom," Hearing before the Tactical Air and Land Forces Subcommittee of the Committee on Armed Services, House of Representatives, One Hundred Ninth Congress, second session: June 15, 2006.

"In his original trial, Dr. Alam measured temperatures of 42 to 44 degrees Celsius": H. B. Alam, Z. Chen, A. Jaskille, R. I. Querol, E. Koustova, R. Inocencio, R. Conran, A. Seufert, et al., "Application of a Zeolite Hemostatic Agent Achieves 100% Survival in a Lethal Model of Complex Groin Injury in Swine." *Journal of Trauma* 56, no. 5, May 2004.

"Subsequent researchers...found a high temperature of 55 degrees Celsius": N. Ahuja, T. A. Ostomel, P. Rhee, G. D. Stucky, R. Conran, Z. Chen, G. A. Al-Mubarak, G. Velmahos, et al., "Testing of Modified Zeolite Hemostatic Dressings in a Large Animal Model of Lethal Groin Injury." *Journal of Trauma* 61, no. 6, Dec. 2006.

"Researchers at Zhejiang University in China—who might be the most objective, because presumably they had no skin in the game": J. Shentu, X. Zhang, J. Fan, "Hemostatic Efficiency and Wound Healing Properties of Natural Zeolite Granules in a Lethal Rabbit Model of Complex Groin Injury." *Materials* 5, no. 12, Dec. 3, 2012.

"The highest temperature was recorded by the Naval Medical Research Center, which found a peak temperature of 70 degrees Celsius": F. Arnaud, T. Tomori, W. Carr, A. McKeague, K. Teranishi, K. Prusaczyk, R. McCarron, "Exothermic Reaction in Zeolite Hemostatic Dressings: QuikClot ACS and ACS+." *Annals of Biomedical Engineering* 36, no. 10, Oct. 2008:1708–1713.

"Using a different model than Dr. Alam had employed, they inflicted wounds to the pigs' livers rather than their femoral arteries and measured a temperature of 100 degrees Celsius": Anthony Pusateri, Angel Delgado, Edward Dick, Raul Martinez, John Holcomb, and Kathy Ryan, "Application of a Granular Mineral-Based Hemostatic Agent (QuikClot) to Reduce Blood Loss After Grade V Liver Injury in Swine." *Journal of Trauma* 57, no. 3, discussion 562, Sept. 2004: 555–62.

"'In practice, burns [produced by QuikClot] were not really a problem'": Robert Little, "Stanching Wounds." *Baltimore Sun*, Nov. 20, 2005.

"When the study was eventually published, it cited temperatures in excess of 95 degrees Celsius": J. K. Wright, J. Kalns, E. A. Wolf, F. Traweek, S. Schwarz, C. K. Loeffler, W. Snyder, L. D. Yantis Jr., et al., "Thermal Injury Resulting from Application of a Granular Mineral Hemostatic Agent." *Journal of Trauma* 57, no. 2, August 2004.

"The navy surgeon Peter Rhee examined 103 cases of QuikClot use in real-world settings": P. Rhee, C. Brown, M. Martin, A. Salim, D. Plurad, D. Green, L. Chambers, et al., "QuikClot Use in Trauma for Hemorrhage Control: Case Series of 103 Documented Uses." *Journal of Trauma* 64, no. 4, April 2008:1093–9.

"'I don't think we want that on our soldiers'": "Special Operations Surgeon Uses Lessons Learned in Somalia to Revolutionize Combat Casualty Care in the Global War on Terrorism" and "Innovations in Hemorrhage Control and Transfusion Paradigms Redefining Trauma Combat Casualty Care Guidelines," Parts 1 and 2, *WarDocs—The Military Medicine Podcast.*

"'What's worse, giving your buddy a little burn while you save his life or doing nothing and letting him die?'": Robert Little, "Stanching Wounds." *Baltimore Sun*, Nov. 20, 2005.

"The War Department and President McKinley gave Langley a $50,000 grant": David Kindy, "This Odd Early Flying Machine Made History but Didn't Have the Right Stuff." *Smithsonian Magazine*, May 5, 2021.

"'like a handful of mortar'": "Lessons from the First Airplane (Long Version)," Lawrence W. Reed, Mackinac Center for Public Policy, July 15, 2003. https://www.mackinac.org/5539

"'You tell Langley for me . . . that the only thing he ever made fly was government money'": Lee Habeeb and Mike Leven, "A Tale of 'Government Investment.'" *National Review*, April 9, 2013.

"It was only when foreign governments were on the verge of working with the Wright brothers": "Starting the Business," Library of Congress, https://www.loc.gov/collections/wilbur-and-orville-wright-papers/articles-and-essays/collection-highlights/starting-the-business/ (Original source: Wilbur and Orville Wright Papers. Library of Congress.)

"At the start of the war, the army favored the M-16 rifle . . . a World War II weapon that appeared unsuited for jungle warfare": James Fallows, "M-16: A Bureaucratic Horror Story." *Atlantic*, June 1981.

"'QuikClot converted wounds that were 100 percent fatal into wounds that were 100 percent nonfatal'": Gina Kolata, "A Nation at War." *New York Times*, March 3, 2003.

"'one of the Iraq war's most dramatic lifesaving technologies'": Melissa Healy, "Lifesaving Product of the War." *Los Angeles Times*, June 23, 2003.

"QuikClot induces the 'rapid coagulation of wounds'": Rome Neal, "High-Tech Medicine on Battlefield." CBS News, March 31, 2003. https://www.cbsnews.com/news/high-tech-medicine-on-battlefield/

"the product 'stems even severe arterial bleeding'": "Cut and Dried." *Economist*, July 24, 2003. https://www.economist.com/science-and-technology/2003/07/24/cut-and-dried

"In its November 2003 issue, *Scientific American* named Francis X. Hursey among its top 50 'research leaders of the year'": The Scientific American 50 List of Winners. *Scientific American*, Nov. 10, 2003. https://www.scientificamerican.com/article/the-2003-scientific-ameri/

"it did have the benefit of providing antibacterial properties, reducing the risk of infections": Marcia Meier, "UCSB Chemistry Professor Wins Top Military Award for Life-Saving Gauze." *UC Santa Barbara Current*, August 11, 2008.

CHAPTER EIGHT: THE DANGER OF USING A SLEDGEHAMMER TO CRACK A NUT

"But Lufkin had told his parents they should not worry because his vehicle was so well protected": Robert Little, "Don't Let Me Die." *Baltimore Sun*, Nov. 20, 2006.

"During his senior year, he'd hit the home run that won Knoxville High School the conference title": "Knoxville Honors Fallen Soldier Caleb Lufkin with Tree, Monument Dedication." WGIL.com, April 23, 2006. https://www.wgil.com/2016/04/23/knoxville-honors-fallen-soldier-caleb-lufkin-with-tree-monument-dedication/

"He also played the banjo, fished, hunted, and rode motorcycles": "Caleb Lufkin Obituary," Legacy.com, from *Peoria Journal Star*, May 31, 2006. https://www.legacy.com/us/obituaries/pjstar/name/caleb-lufkin-obituary?id=29936884

"Just before noon on May 4, the last thing that Lufkin saw before the improvised explosive device went off under the truck was a boy riding a bicycle": Robert Little, "Don't Let Me Die." *Baltimore Sun*, Nov. 20, 2006.

"Caleb Lufkin's arrival at the combat hospital was captured by a CNN camera crew": *CNN Presents: Combat Hospital* (2006). Vimeo. https://vimeo.com/32419849

"When Lufkin arrived at the triage room at the Tenth Combat Support Hospital, the surgeon, David Steinbruner, said to him": Ibid.

"Lufkin said, 'Caleb.' . . . 'Breathe deep for me, Caleb' ": Ibid.

"As commander of the Institute of Surgical Research, he largely had carte blanche to go in and out of Iraq and Afghanistan as he chose": "Special Operations Surgeon Uses Lessons Learned in Somalia to Revolutionize Combat Casualty Care in the Global War on Terrorism" and "Innovations in Hemorrhage Control and Transfusion Paradigms Redefining Trauma Combat Casualty Care Guidelines," Parts 1 and 2, *WarDocs—The Military Medicine Podcast.*

" 'His blood pressure was eighty, he'd lost about forty percent of his blood volume' ": Robert Little, "Don't Let Me Die." *Baltimore Sun*, Nov. 20, 2006.

"Hemophilia, a serious blood clotting disorder, is an extremely rare condition": "The A's and B's of Hemophilia," Pfizer. https://www.pfizer.com/news/articles/'s-and-b's-hemophilia

"Factor Seven worked by increasing the amount of the seventh factor of the body's clotting system as much as a thousandfold": Harold R. Roberts, Dougald M. Monroe, and Gilbert C. White, "The Use of Recombinant Factor VIIa in the Treatment of Bleeding Disorders." *Blood* 104, no. 13, 2004.

"Factor Seven, at $5,000 or more a dose, was one of the costliest drugs in the world": Bernard Wysocki, " 'Wonder Drug' Stops Bleeding, but Cost Is High." *Wall Street Journal*, March 17, 2004.

"would Factor Seven create clots not only at the wound site, but also in the wrong places—in the heart and lungs and brain—where they could

cause heart attacks and strokes": Robert Little, "Dangerous Remedy." *Baltimore Sun*, Nov. 19, 2006.

"Three weeks after receiving Factor Seven during his operation in Baghdad, Caleb Lufkin died of cardiac arrest": Robert Little, "Don't Let Me Die." *Baltimore Sun*, Nov. 20, 2006.

"'The worst feeling in a physician's life is when you are just standing there'": Robert Little, "Dubious Breakthrough." *Baltimore Sun*, Nov. 21, 2006.

"they left the conference agreeing that a newly introduced drug, Factor Seven, had great potential to be the next candidate": Ibid.

"'The hemophiliacs who were inpatients at the medical clinic'": U. K. Hedner, *Treating Life-Threatening Bleedings: Development of Recombinant Coagulation Factor VIIa* (Elsevier, 2017), 15.

"'It was so clear that the patients with hemophilia...were so lousily treated'": "MeetTheHERO: MD PhD Ulla Hedner, pioneer in haemophilia treatment," Novo Nordisk, MP4, 1:28. https://video.novonordisk.com/video /11478324/meetthehero-md-phd-ulla-hedner-pioneer

"'This tragic event occurred...when I was working as laboratory technician'": Hedner, *Life-Threatening Bleedings*, 15.

"However, a small subset of patients, perhaps 10 percent, have inhibitors": "Inhibitors and Hemophilia," Centers for Disease Control and Prevention. https://www.cdc.gov/ncbddd/hemophilia/inhibitors.html

"Upon receiving Factor Seven, the patient recovered more quickly than expected": Hedner, *Life-Threatening Bleedings*, 22.

"today Novo Nordisk produces half of the world's insulin supply": Bill Berkrot, "Novo Nordisk to Supply Insulin at Discount to Poorest Nations." Reuters, Sept. 21, 2016. https://www.reuters.com/article/us-novo-nordisk-diabetes/novo-nordisk-to -supply-insulin-at-discount-to-poorest-nations-idUSKCN11R2X2; F. Kansteiner, "Lawmakers Blast Pharma for 'Outrageous' Prices and 'Anticompetitive Conduct' in Culmination of 3-Year Probe." *Fierce Pharma*, Dec. 10, 2021.

"Factor Seven be cloned and introduced into the kidney cells of baby hamsters": "NovoSeven Coagulation Factor VIIa (Recombinant)," United States Food and Drug Administration. https://www.fda.gov/media/70435/download

"Hedner heard of the Orphan Drug Act only by pure happenstance": Hedner, *Life-Threatening Bleedings*, 45.

"Remarkably, seven of the ten best-selling drugs in the United States in 2015 originated as orphan drugs": Sarah Jane Tribble and Sydney Lupkin, "Drugs for Rare Diseases Have Become Uncommonly Rich Monopolies," Jan. 17, 2017, in *Morning Edition*, produced by NPR, radio program, MP3, 5:26. https://www.npr .org/sections/health-shots/2017/01/17/509506836/drugs-for-rare-diseases-have become-uncommonly-rich-monopolies

"'Now, another thing about Factor Seven, it provoked a whole school of thinking'": "The CONTROL trial: Factor VIIa in Trauma—Podcast #4," Sept. 14, 2011, in *Traumacast*, produced by the Eastern Association for the Surgery of Trauma, podcast, MP3, 36:00. https://www.east.org/education-career-development/online-education /traumacasts/detail/9/the-control-trial-factor-viia-in-trauma

"At the time of the incident, Martinowitz was planning to conduct a trial of Factor Seven on pigs": Robert Little, "Dubious Breakthrough." *Baltimore Sun*, Nov. 21, 2006.

"Published only five months after the incident, the article does not read like a typical medical journal article": G. Kenet, R. Walden, A. Eldad, and U. Martinowitz, "Treatment of Traumatic Bleeding with Recombinant Factor VIIa." *Lancet* 354, no. 9193, Nov. 27, 1999: 1879.

"The *Lancet* is arguably the world's leading medical journal": "About the *Lancet*: Reach and Impact," https://www.thelancet.com/lancet/about

"'It's got incredible potential,' Vandre said": Jessica Marshall, "Saved by Sand Poured into Wounds." *New Scientist*, March 15, 2006. https://www.newscientist.com /article/mg18925435-800-saved-by-sand-poured-into-the-wounds/

"This forced Novo Nordisk to conduct the trial outside of the United States": Robert Little, "Dubious Breakthrough." *Baltimore Sun*, Nov. 21, 2006.

"The results of the study were published in the *Journal of Trauma* and appeared to report positive outcomes": K. D. Boffard, B. Riou, B. Warren, P. I. Choong, S. Rizoli, R. Rossaint, M. Axelsen, et al., "Recombinant Factor VIIa as Adjunctive Therapy for Bleeding Control in Severely Injured Trauma Patients: Two Parallel Randomized, Placebo-Controlled, Double-Blind Clinical Trials." *Journal of Trauma* 59, no. 1, 2005.

"Hematologists Kathryn Webert and Morris Blajchman of McMaster University in Canada accused the researchers of 'information laundering'": K. E Webert, M. A. Blajchman, "Randomized Trials in Patients with Blunt and Penetrating Trauma," *Journal of Trauma* 60, no. 1, Jan. 2006: 242–3; author reply 243–4.

"'When it works, it's amazing'": Robert Little, "Dangerous Remedy." *Baltimore Sun*, Nov. 19, 2006.

"As a doctor who worked under Holcomb, and who would later challenge the army's use of Factor Seven in a whistleblower lawsuit": Sig Christensen and Don Finley, "Drug Firm's Wooing Made Whistleblower Suspicious." *San Antonio Express-News*, June 26, 2011. https://www.mysanantonio.com/news/military /article/Drug-firm-s-wooing-made-whistleblower-suspicious-1440664.php

"A significant part of the American military budget is spent on pharmaceutical drugs": J. Schwartz, "Soaring Cost of Military Drugs Could Hurt Budget." *Austin American-Statesman*, Dec. 29, 2012.

"John Holcomb formally made the decision to move forward with Factor Seven as a standard treatment for bleeding soldiers in Iraq in February 2004": Robert Little, "Dangerous Remedy." *Baltimore Sun*, Nov. 19, 2006.

"The drug arrived at army combat hospitals shortly thereafter, in early 2004": Robert Little, "Untested in Battle." *Baltimore Sun*, March 29, 2009.

"The army's guidelines were liberal, allowing doctors to inject the drug before it was clear that patients were suffering life-threatening hemorrhage": Robert Little, "Dubious Breakthrough." *Baltimore Sun*, Nov. 21, 2006.

"'Army protocol in Baghdad called for injecting it into virtually every casualty with signs of serious bleeding'": Robert Little, "Drugmaker Pays $25 Million to Settle Military Claim." *Baltimore Sun*, June 10, 2011.

"'When you give a patient a powerful clot-promoting medication, you may well induce a clot some place you don't want one'": Robert Little, "Don't Let Me Die." *Baltimore Sun*, Nov. 20, 2006.

"'It's a completely irresponsible and inappropriate use of a very, very dangerous drug'": Robert Little, "Dangerous Remedy." *Baltimore Sun*, Nov. 19, 2006.

"military surgeons observed 'startling' rates of blood clots in the lungs and veins of soldiers": A. Gawande, "Casualties of War—Military Care for the Wounded from Iraq and Afghanistan." *New England Journal of Medicine* 351, no. 24, Dec. 9, 2004.

"'We see some strokes,' said another doctor": Robert Little, "Dangerous Remedy." *Baltimore Sun*, Nov. 19, 2006.

"'It's insane, using it that way. Absolutely insane'": Robert Little, "Dangerous Remedy." *Baltimore Sun*, Nov. 19, 2006.

"'British Soldiers Are "Guinea Pigs"'": O. Dyer, "British Soldiers Are 'Guinea Pigs' for New Use of Blood Clotting Agent." *British Medical Journal*, Sept. 23, 2006.

"'his efforts, however well intended, may be doing more harm than good'": Alex Berenson, "Army's Aggressive Surgeon Too Aggressive for Some." *New York Times*, Nov. 6, 2007.

"'In managing bleeding, we must not use a sledgehammer to crack a nut'": V. Tarzia, E. Buratto, G. Bortolussi, C. Paolini, J. Bejko, T. Bottio, and G. Gerosa, "The Danger of Using a Sledgehammer to Crack a Nut: ROTEM-Guided Administration of Recombinant Activated Factor VII in a Patient with Refractory Bleeding Post-Ventricular Assist Device Implantation." *Artificial Organs* 39, no. 3, March 2015.

"'Of course some of them are dying from it'": Robert Little, "Dangerous Remedy." *Baltimore Sun*, Nov. 19, 2006.

"Even though Holcomb, as the *New York Times* wrote, 'understood the concerns of the Army's critics and agreed there was no strong evidence that the drug decreases mortality or other complications in trauma patients'": Alex Berenson, "Army's Aggressive Surgeon Too Aggressive for Some." *New York Times*, Nov. 6, 2007.

"'To say that because you're in a war, everything you do is right, suggests to me a level of arrogance that can only lead to a poor outcome'": Robert Little, "Dangerous Remedy." *Baltimore Sun*, Nov. 19, 2006.

"'If you've got young soldiers having weirdo strokes'": Siri Nilsson, "Dangerous Gamble." *ABC News*, Dec. 5, 2006. https://abcnews.go.com/Health/story?id=2693934&page=1

"'You can't conduct clinical research in the middle of a war,' he said in 2006": Robert Little, "Dubious Breakthrough." *Baltimore Sun*, Nov. 21, 2006.

"'We've been tracking patient outcomes as best we can'": Siri Nilsson, "Dangerous Gamble." *ABC News*, Dec. 5, 2006.

"When it came to Factor Seven, Holcomb said, 'We're not waiting' for more clinical research": Robert Little, "Dangerous Remedy." *Baltimore Sun*, Nov. 19, 2006.

"Serious adverse events occurred in 2 percent of the placebo-treated patients, compared to 7 percent of the Factor Seven–treated patients":

S. A. Mayer, N. C. Brun, K. Begtrup, J. Broderick, S. Davis, M. N. Diringer, B. E. Skolnick, et al., "Recombinant Activated Factor VII Intracerebral Hemorrhage Trial Investigators." *New England Journal of Medicine* 352, no. 8, Feb. 24, 2005.

"The warning was included in the package insert for the product": K. A. O'Connell, J. J. Wood, R. P. Wise, J. N. Lozier, M. M. Braun, "Thromboembolic Adverse Events after Use of Recombinant Human Coagulation Factor VIIa." *JAMA* 295, no. 3, Jan. 18, 2006.

"The researchers reviewed adverse events after administration of Factor Seven that were reported to the FDA between 1999 and 2004": Ibid.

"It found an 8.7 percent rate of clot-related complications, which included twelve deaths partially attributed to the drug": Robert Little, "Factor Seven Timeline." *Baltimore Sun*, Nov. 19, 2006.

"They noted that one-third of the complications that patients had experienced were associated with the drug itself, a percentage which the British doctors found 'highly consistent' with other large Factor Seven trials": T. J. Hodgetts, E. Kirkman, P. F. Mahoney, R. Russell, R. Thomas, M. Midwinter, "UK Defence Medical Services Guidance for the Use of Recombinant Factor VIIa (rFVIIa) in the Deployed Military Setting." *Journal of the Royal Army Medical Corps* 153, no. 4, Dec. 2007.

" 'In the 14 years Factor Seven has been clinically used, only a few cases of myocardial infarction [heart attack] and stroke have occurred' ": J. B. Holcomb, "Use of Recombinant Activated Factor VII to Treat the Acquired Coagulopathy of Trauma." *Journal of Trauma* 58, no. 6, June 2005.

" 'You have a drug you know is safe from the prospective randomized controlled clinical trials' ": Alex Berenson, "Army's Aggressive Surgeon Too Aggressive for Some." *New York Times*, Nov. 6, 2007.

"prescriptions for Factor Seven increased more than 140 times": A. C. Logan, V. Yank, and R. S. Stafford, "Off-Label Use of Recombinant Factor VIIa in U.S. Hospitals: Analysis of Hospital Records." *Annals of Internal Medicine* 154, no. 8, April 19, 2011.

"By 2008, people with hemophilia accounted for only 3 percent of the drug's in-hospital use, while an extraordinary 97 percent of its use was for off-label indications": André Côté and Bernard Keating, "What Is Wrong with Orphan Drug Policies?" *Value in Health* 15, no. 8, 2012.

"Holcomb had pushed aggressively for the use of a new, lightweight tourniquet": Robert Little, "Modern Combat Lacking in Old Medical Supply." *Baltimore Sun*, March 6, 2005.

"the army responded by sending an additional 172,000 new-generation tourniquets to its soldiers": Robert Little, "US Military Widening Use of Tourniquets." *Baltimore Sun*, May 2, 2005.

"light up a room at social events": Dennis Owens, "Widener Remembers Fallen Alum with Scholarship." ABC27.com, Nov. 11, 2016. https://www.abc27.com/news/widener-law-remembers-fallen-alum-with-scholarship/

"Mahaffee, who had thick dark hair and a rugged athletic build, had served in the army reserves as a young man and retired in 1999": Robert Little, "Don't Let Me Die." *Baltimore Sun*, Nov. 20, 2006.

" 'He was talking about setting up a security perimeter when one of the enlisted men' ": "3rd Annual Captain Shane Mahaffee Memorial," Golf Digest Planner. https://www.planmygolfevent.com/6670-3rd_Annual_Captain_Mahaffee/Photos.html

" 'He needs it,' one of the attending physicians said, 'because he's going to bleed like hell.' " Robert Little, "Don't Let Me Die." *Baltimore Sun*, Nov. 20, 2006.

" 'With these poly-trauma patients, once they start to get oozy, they can just spiral downhill. You can't wait for that to happen' ": Ibid.

"but as Robert Little later wrote, 'His doctors said it was the ventilator that likely prompted the infection' ": Ibid.

" 'I had a very bad feeling about his injury from the beginning,' said Mahaffee's widow": Ibid.

" 'It's paid with American blood' ": Dennis Owens, "Widener Remembers Fallen Alum with Scholarship." ABC27.com, Nov. 11, 2016.

" 'Try to imagine walking through that door and seeing your perfect child lying there' ": Robert Little, "Don't Let Me Die." *Baltimore Sun*, Nov. 20, 2006.

" 'After what these kids did for us, we can't even give them a clean room to recover in?' ": Robert Little, "Flawed Jewel." *Baltimore Sun*, March 11, 2007.

" 'He was starting to finally come to life' ": Robert Little, "Don't Let Me Die." *Baltimore Sun*, Nov. 20, 2006.

" 'No one's ever been able to explain to me how someone so young and so healthy could die of a heart attack like that' ": Ibid.

"His army autopsy reported only that Lufkin had perished of complications of injuries from a bomb blast": Ibid.

" 'I can't bring my kid back but maybe we can get somebody to take responsibility' ": Marcus Baram, "Go to War, Serve Your Country, Become a Guinea Pig?" KTRE.com, Dec. 7, 2006. https://www.ktre.com/story/5782326/go-to-war-serve-your-country-become-a-guinea-pig/

" 'You can't keep pushing the buck on somebody else' ": Ibid.

"A group of protesters from Westboro held signs, and children and teens sang, 'Filthy fags, God hates you' ": Tom Loewy, "Tom Loewy: Keep Wall between Church and State High." *State Journal-Register*, May 7, 2010. https://www.sj-r.com/story/news/2010/05/07/tom-loewy-keep-wall-between/48297547007/

" 'He died for that flag' ": Robert Little, "Don't Let Me Die." *Baltimore Sun*, Nov. 20, 2006.

"in 2014 the tree was unintentionally cut down during construction at the school": "Illinois School Cuts Down Tree Honoring Dead Soldier." NBC Chicago, April 8, 2014. https://www.nbcchicago.com/news/national-international/knoxville-illinois-tree-caleb-lufkin/1976847/

"a new oak tree was planted, and an engraved granite memorial dedicated to Lufkin": Elizabeth Wadas, "Small Town Hero Honored 10 Years after Death." WQAD.com, April 23, 2016. https://www.wqad.com/article/news/local/drone

/8-in-the-air/small-town-hero-honored-10-years-after-death/526-5ff941c5-f6e6
-47af-94d0-49f823b119be

CHAPTER NINE: EMOTIONAL BANKRUPTCY

"defense industry publication reported that QuikClot had saved 150 lives in Iraq and Afghanistan by 2006": "Army 'Rapid Equipping Force' Taking Root, Chief Says." *National Defense*, Oct. 1, 2006. https://www.nationalde fensemagazine.org/articles/2006/10/1/2006october-army-rapid-equipping-force -taking-root-chief-says

"the number of Iraqi deaths, astoundingly, had been about thirty times greater than those suffered by the US military": "Costs of War. Iraqi Civilians," June 2021. Watson Institute, International and Public Affairs, Brown University. https://watson.brown.edu/costsofwar/costs/human/civilians/iraqi

CHAPTER TEN: *UNITED STATES V. NOVO NORDISK*

" 'I urge you to immediately review the use and effects of this drug' ": "Mikulski Demands Answers on Report That Battlefield Drug Puts Soldiers at Risk." *Southern Maryland Online*, Nov. 29, 2006. http://somd.com/news/headlines/2006 /4898.php

" 'The safety of our troops is the top priority' ": Robert Little, "Senators Seek Review of Blood Drug's Use," *Los Angeles Times*, Nov. 30, 2006.

" 'At no time have we seen increases in complications' ": John Holcomb, "Recombinant Factor VIIa (rFVIIa) History, Use in Civilian Trauma, Combat Operations, Complications and Outcomes" to Defense Subcommittee of the Senate Appropriations Committee. Dec 7, 2006.

"at the same hospital in 2008, it was used a dozen times in six months": Robert Little, "Untested in Battle." *Baltimore Sun*, March 29, 2009.

"the British military essentially stopped using Factor Seven": T. J. Hodgetts, E. Kirkman, P. F. Mahoney, R. Russell, R. Thomas, and M. Midwinter, "UK Defence Medical Services Guidance for the Use of Recombinant Factor VIIa (rFVIIa) in the Deployed Military Setting." *Journal of the Royal Army Medical Corps*, 2007.

"Demetriades captured the entire Factor Seven story with the following pithy anecdote": D. Demetriades, MD, PhD, FACS, "Trauma: From Inception to Date— Successes, Trials, Errors and Challenges" (presentation, WVU School of Medicine Department of Surgery, 2016).

"colleagues accused Holcomb of 'initiating numerous and consistent actions of mismanagement and misuse of authority and funding associated within his function' ": Letter to the Office of the Inspector General, RE: Behavior in Violation of Federal Policy and Regulation, March 12, 2007.

"The writers pointed out that Holcomb had recommended HemCon for use on the battlefield despite unpublished studies": Ibid.

"colleagues' concerns that the Institute of Surgical Research under Holcomb 'stressed results at the expense of good science'": Memorandum for COL Blackbourne, Commander USAISR. Subject: Issues of Research Misconduct at US-AISR, December 3, 2008.

"as both 'arrogant, obnoxious, [and] overbearing' and 'exactly the type of leader the ISR needed'": Robert Little, "Untested in Battle." *Baltimore Sun*, March 29, 2009.

"stress of the investigation": Ibid.

"Holcomb was awarded a medal reserved for those who have made outstanding contributions to special operations": Committee on Tactical Combat Casualty Care Meeting Minutes July 22–24, 2008. https://www.jsomonline.org/TCCCEsp/04%20Resumen%20de%20las%20Reuniones%20del%20CoTCCC%20(en%20ingles)/CoTCCC%20Meeting%20Minutes%2008 07%20Final.pdf

"'We've been able to reduce the number of trauma deaths at our hospital by thirty percent just by applying the skills I learned in the military'": Ramin A. Khalili, "Resuscitation, Retro Style: Saving Lives with Whole Blood." *DC Military*, Oct. 14, 2016. https://www.dcmilitary.com/standard/news/resuscitation-retro-style-saving-lives-with-whole-blood/article_fdf46e84-7bfc-5f96-b985-6f0835baaeab.html

"Dr. Black filed the complaint on the day of his resignation because he feared retaliation from his former superiors": Sig Christensen and Don Finley, "Drug Firm's Wooing Made Whistleblower Suspicious." *San Antonio Express-News*, June 26, 2011.

"tuition paid for by the army": I. Black, "The War Goes On." *JAMA* 300, no. 11, Sept. 17, 2008.

"'a cornucopia of pain'": Melissa Block, "Army Burn Center Sees Some of Worst War Wounds," July 20, 2006, in *All Things Considered*, produced by NPR, radio program, MP3, 12:56.

"Black said, 'They asked me if I used the drug. I said yes. They said, "Good, you're an expert."'": Sig Christensen and Don Finley, "Army Again Probing Fort Sam Payments." *San Antonio Express-News*, June 14, 2011.

"'oh my God, these guys are playing me,' he said": Sig Christensen and Don Finley, "Drug Firm's Wooing Made Whistleblower Suspicious." *San Antonio Express-News*, June 26, 2011.

"'was tired beyond words'": Ian Black, "Working with the Wounded: Tired, But Not Numb," Dec. 26, 2006, in *All Things Considered*, produced by NPR, radio program, MP3, 5:19. https://www.npr.org/2006/12/26/6682412/working-with-the-wounded-tired-but-not-numb

"The injuries were horrific": Ibid.

"The clogs he wore in the operating room had become rotten from the amount of time he'd spent standing in blood": Ian H. Black, "A Boring Thanksgiving." *Anesthesiology* 117, no. 5, Nov. 2012.

"Eventually, he had to wear galoshes": "Working with the Wounded," Dec. 26, 2006, in *All Things Considered*.

"'Don't worry, Mama, it was only a leg. I'll be all right'": I. Black, "The War Goes On." *JAMA* 300, no. 11, 2008.

"Black said, 'It didn't mean for sure it caused it, but it certainly gave me pause'": Sig Christensen and Don Finley, "Drug Firm's Wooing Made Whistleblower Suspicious." *San Antonio Express-News*, June 26, 2011.

"Black was ordered to do a study of clinical practice guidelines": Ibid.

"the survival rate of patients in their hospital remained the same after this dramatic reduction": Ibid.

"Holcomb agreed": Ibid.

"contractors sold sick horses and mules, malfunctioning rifles, and spoiled provisions to the Union Army": "Government Contractor & Procurement Fraud," Waters Kraus & Paul. https://waterskraus.com/practice-areas/qui-tam -whistleblower/procurement-fraud/

"Parke-Davis paid $430 million in fines to the government, and Franklin himself received $24 million": United States Department of Justice, "Warner-Lambert to Pay $430 Million to Resolve Criminal & Civil Health Care Liability Relating to Off-Label Promotion," May 13, 2004. https://www.justice.gov/archive /opa/pr/2004/May/04_civ_322.htm

"Novo Nordisk illegally funded medical experiments on injured soldiers in Iraq in order to widen the use of Factor Seven. In fact, experimenting on soldiers injured in battle is illegal. Only the US president is able to sign a waiver that allows research drugs to be used on American soldiers": "Drug Company Illegally Experimented on Wounded Soldiers in Iraq," Jim Edwards, CBS News, July 5, 2011. https://www.cbsnews.com/news/drug-company -illegally-experimented-on-wounded-soldiers-in-iraq-suit-says/

"Novo Nordisk promoted Factor Seven to US Army doctors and researchers at the Institute of Surgical Research, which included John Holcomb": John Tedesco, "Military Medicine Scheme Is Alleged." *San Antonio Express-News*, July 16, 2011.

"the payment of speaker, conference, and research fees that functioned as kickbacks": "Drug Company Illegally Experimented on Wounded Soldiers in Iraq," CBS News, July 5, 2011.

"The suit references twenty examples of Novo Nordisk sponsoring studies, seminars, trips, meals, and honoraria for army physicians from 2005 to 2007 ... given meals at New York Prime, a four-star steakhouse, and Emeril's, another high-end restaurant": Ibid; "Military Medicine Scheme Is Alleged." *San Antonio Express-News*, July 16, 2011.

"They were given, for example, a trip on the *Queen Elizabeth 2* to visit Novo Nordisk's collection of castles in Denmark": Ibid.

"It is, however, illegal for a company outside the government to pay inducements to federal employees": Ibid.

"Army physicians are required to follow federal laws and military regulations that generally prohibit honoraria and many types of gifts from third parties": "Military Medicine Scheme Is Alleged." *San Antonio Express-News*, July 16, 2011.

"'money-laundering device through which Novo [Nordisk] funneled cash to military doctors willing to promote the use of [Factor Seven] to their colleagues'": "Drug Company Illegally Experimented on Wounded Soldiers in Iraq," CBS News, July 5, 2011.

"The lawsuit goes on to describe the T.R.U.E. foundation as a 'sham' organization": "Military Medicine Scheme Is Alleged." *San Antonio Express-News*, July 16, 2011.

"Indeed the initials in the T.R.U.E. acronym didn't actually stand for anything... 'Hell, if they needed a new computer, we could buy them a new computer'": Ibid.

"He returned at least two more times": John Tedesco, "Military Medicine Scheme Is Alleged." *San Antonio Express-News*, July 20, 2011.

"In 2009 the gross receipts of the T.R.U.E. foundation, whose stated mission was 'improving the quality of military medicine through research and education,' were about $13 million": T.R.U.E. Research Foundation, 990 Filing, Department of the Treasury, Internal Revenue Service. https://pdf.guidestar.org/PDF_Images/2010/742/855/2010-742855021-06c98bbb-9.pdf?_gl=1*ylk1ol*_ga*MTYxMTE2OTk4Ni4xNjY4NzM5MDcy*_ga_5W8PXYYGBX*MTY3MDkwMDA5NC4yLjEuMTY3MDkwMDIzMS41MS4wLjA.&_ga=2.64070831.1845004516.1670900095-1611169986.1668739072

"Bordas and Nakamura frequently clashed and that the foundation's board was unhappy with their spending habits": John Tedesco, "Military Medicine Scheme Is Alleged." *San Antonio Express-News*, July 20, 2011.

"added a warning to the label": V. Yank, C. V. Tuohy, A. C. Logan, et al. Comparative Effectiveness of In-Hospital Use of Recombinant Factor VIIa for Off-Label Indications vs. Usual Care [Internet]. Rockville (MD): Agency for Healthcare Research and Quality (US); 2010 May. (Comparative Effectiveness Reviews, No. 21.) Introduction.

CHAPTER ELEVEN: THE ARMY'S GREATEST INVENTION

"They tested kaolin against the original granular QuikClot and discovered that it worked just as well, but without any of the large heat release": Adrian Castaneda, "UCSB Research Improves Blood-Clotting Gauze." *Santa Barbara Independent*, August 14, 2008.

"the nanoparticles of kaolin congregated at the wound site, and did not enter the circulatory system": Aaron Rowe, "Nanoparticles Help Gauze Stop Gushing Wounds." *Wired*, April 24, 2008. https://www.wired.com/2008/04/nanoparticles-help-gauze-stop-gushing-wounds/

"approximate 90 percent effectiveness": Yuval Ran, Eran Hadad, Saleh Daher, Ori Ganor, Jonathan Kohn, Yana Yegorov, Carmi Bartal, Nachman Ash, and Gil Hirschhorn, "QuikClot Combat Gauze Use for Hemorrhage Control in Military Trauma: January 2009 Israel Defense Force Experience in the Gaza Strip—a Preliminary Report of 14 Cases." *Prehospital and Disaster Medicine*, Nov.–Dec. 2010.

"The navy and Marine Corps then gave Z-Medica almost $3 million to conduct human studies of the kaolin": Z-Medica Corp., "Z-Medica Awarded $2.9 Million US Navy/Marine Corp Contract for Penetrating Wound Study Using its New Hemostatic Gauze," Oct. 13, 2008. https://www.prweb.com/releases/2008/10/prweb1446784.htm

"recommended 'Combat Gauze as the first-line treatment for life-threatening hemorrhage that is not amenable to tourniquet placement'": Minutes of the Committee on Tactical Combat Casualty Care, Institute of Surgical Research, April 1–2, 2008. https://www.jsomonline.org/TCCC/03%20CoTCCC%20Meeting%20Minutes/CoTCCC%20Meeting%20Minutes%200804.pdf

"The army alone bought 270,000 packages of Combat Gauze": RDECOM Public Affairs, Sarah Maxwell, "Army Medicine Improves with New Dressings." United States Army, Oct. 17, 2008. https://www.army.mil/article/13413/army_medicine_improves_with_new_dressings

"Stucky said, 'I am very honored'": Marcia Meier, "UCSB Chemistry Professor Wins Top Military Award for Life-Saving Gauze." *UC Santa Barbara Current*, August 11, 2008.

"Its developer was identified as the 'U.S. Army Institute of Surgical Research,' and Z-Medica was not mentioned at all": RDECOM Public Affairs, "U.S. Army Recognizes Top Ten Greatest Inventions of 2008." United States Army, Sept. 18, 2009. https://www.army.mil/article/27563/u_s_army_recognizes_top_ten_greatest_inventions_of_2008

"Black and Montiel received about $3.5 million each": Sig Christensen and Don Finley, "Army Again Probing Fort Sam Payments." *San Antonio Express-News*, June 14, 2011.

"The Department of Justice's press release stated": United States Department of Justice, "Danish Pharmaceutical Novo Nordisk to Pay $25 Million to Resolve Allegations of Off-Label Promotion of Novoseven," June 10, 2011. https://www.justice.gov/opa/pr/danish-pharmaceutical-novo-nordisk-pay-25-million-resolve-allegations-label-promotion

"filed for bankruptcy in June 2011": John Tedesco, "Military Medicine Scheme Is Alleged." *San Antonio Express-News*, July 20, 2011.

"'You couldn't get a more graphic example of why there should be much more criminal prosecutions of companies like this'": Ibid.

"'You know, I was wined and dined by the companies'": Ibid.

"'I wasn't trying to assign blame or to make money, I just wanted it to stop'": Robert Little, "Drugmaker Pays $25 Million to Settle Military Claim." *Baltimore Sun*, June 10, 2011.

"'Did I hurt someone?'": Robert Little, "Untested in Battle." *Baltimore Sun*, March 29, 2009.

"'John Holcomb's six years of leadership at the...helm were transformational'": Lorne H. Blackbourne and Basil Pruitt Jr., "The Warrior's Combat Surgeon: COL (ret.) John B. Holcomb, MD, FACS—US Army 1985–2008." *Journal of Trauma* 66, no. 4, April 2009.

"'All he cared about was doing what was right by the soldiers and stopping

bleeding'": Sig Christensen and Don Finley, "Drug Firm's Wooing Made Whistle-blower Suspicious." *San Antonio Express-News*, June 26, 2011.

"In 2014, Holcomb won the Major Jonathan Letterman Medical Excellence Award": "Dr. Holcomb Presented with 2016 Medical Excellence Award," Steven Galvan, United States Army Medical Research and Development Command. https://mrdc.health.mil/index.cfm/media/articles/2016/dr_holcomb_presented_with _2016_medical_excellence_award

" 'There is no one who has been responsible for saving more lives among U.S. casualties in Iraq and Afghanistan than John Holcomb'": Frumentarius, "Combat Surgeon and Special Operations Forces Hero: Dr. John Holcomb." SOFREP, Jan. 1, 2017. https://sofrep.com/news/combat-surgeon-and-special -operations-forces-hero-dr-john-holcomb/

"He played a crucial role in the successful revamping of transportation systems that brought the wounded to appropriate levels of care, which involved a complex collaboration among frontline units, forward surgical teams, and hospitals": Alex Berenson, "Army's Aggressive Surgeon Too Aggressive for Some." *New York Times*, Nov. 6, 2007.

" 'We were all young surgeons and we were doing what we thought was crazy'": George, *Nine Pints*, p. 257.

"Component therapy was considered a state-of-the art, major advance, despite somewhat limited data on its effectiveness": V. T. Ramakrishnan and S. Cattamanchi, "Transfusion Practices in Trauma." *Indian Journal of Anaesthesia* 58, no. 5, 2014.

"transfusing whole blood occurred only in austere environments": S. C. Nessen, B. J. Eastridge, D. Cronk, R. M. Craig, O. Berséus, R. Ellison, K. Remick, J. Seery, A. Shah, P. C. Spinella, "Fresh Whole Blood Use by Forward Surgical Teams in Afghanistan Is Associated with Improved Survival Compared to Component Therapy without Platelets." *Transfusion* 53, Jan. 2013 Supplement.

" 'Blood banks and bedside clinicians all report difficulty with coordinating the preparation, thawing, checking, delivering, and transfusing all these products at the same time and in the correct order'": J. B. Holcomb and D. H. Jenkins, "Get Ready: Whole Blood Is Back and It's Good for Patients." *Transfusion* 58, no. 8, Aug. 2018.

"In massively bleeding patients, he argued, every minute counts": Ibid.

" 'It is NOT appropriate, as a matter of convenience, to use FWB'": Andrew P. Cap, MC USA, Andrew Beckett, MC CAF, Avi Benov, MC IDF, Matthew Borgman, MC USA, Jacob Chen, MC IDF, Jason B. Corley, MSC USA, Heidi Doughty et al., "Whole Blood Transfusion." *Military Medicine* 183, supplement 2, Sept.–Oct. 2018.

"Once again the army began using whole blood": S. C. Nessen, B. J. Eastridge, D. Cronk, R. M. Craig, O. Berséus, R. Ellison, K. Remick, J. Seery, A. Shah, P. C. Spinella, "Fresh Whole Blood Use by Forward Surgical Teams in Afghanistan Is Associated with Improved Survival Compared to Component Therapy without Platelets." *Transfusion* 53, Jan. 2013.

"An international research team did a study in 2010 of twenty thousand trauma patients in forty countries and found that tranexamic acid de-

creased mortality by about 10 percent compared with placebo": H. Shakur, I. Roberts, R. Bautista, et al., "Effects of Tranexamic Acid on Death, Vascular Occlusive Events, and Blood Transfusion in Trauma Patients with Significant Haemorrhage (CRASH-2): A Randomised, Placebo-Controlled Trial." *Lancet* 376, 2010; Ian Roberts, MD, personal correspondence, Nov. 2022.

"It is estimated that the drug could save up to 128,000 of those lives a year, four thousand of them in the United States": Donald G. McNeil Jr., "A Cheap Drug Is Found to Save Bleeding Victims." *New York Times*, March 20, 2012.

"As the *New York Times* wrote in 2012: 'the drug's very inexpensiveness has slowed its entry into American emergency rooms' ": Ibid.

"Siegel's lawsuit accuses Novo Nordisk of attempting to increase profits... Novo Nordisk paid kickbacks to 'anyone who could influence' the prescribing of Factor Seven—including the patient, their family, the physician, and pharmacies": "Doc Alleges Novo Nordisk Ran Kickback Scheme for Hemophilia Drug," Valerie Bauman, Bloomberg Law, May 29, 2020. https://news.bloomberglaw.com/pharma-and-life-sciences/doc-alleges-novo-nordisk -ran-kickback-scheme-for-hemophilia-drug

"Novo Nordisk paid a settlement of $58 million for failure to comply with FDA rules": United States Department of Justice, "Novo Nordisk Agrees to Pay $58 Million for Failure to Comply with FDA-Mandated Risk Program," Sept. 5, 2017.

"The US Congress has also investigated apparent collusion around price increases for insulin products made by three competing companies, including Novo Nordisk": D. Bartz, "Drugmakers Aim Big Price Hikes at U.S. Patients, Congressional Report Finds." Reuters, Dec. 10, 2021. https://www.reuters .com/world/us/drugmakers-aim-big-price-hikes-us-patients-congressional-report -2021-12-10/; F. Kansteiner, "Lawmakers Blast Pharma for 'Outrageous' Prices and 'Anticompetitive Conduct' in Culmination of 3-Year Probe." *Fierce Pharma*, Dec. 10, 2021. https://www.fiercepharma.com/pharma/house-oversight-committee-blasts -pharma-for-outrageous-prices-and-anticompetitive-conduct; F. Kansteiner, Novo Nordisk Comes Out Clean in $1.8B Investor Lawsuit Alleging Insulin Misdirection." *Fierce Pharma*, Jan. 14, 2022. https://www.fiercepharma.com/pharma/novo-nordisk -comes-out-clean-2019-investor-lawsuit-alleging-insulin-misdirection; Bernard Sanders and Elijah E. Cummings to Loretta E. Lynch and Edith Ramirez, Nov. 3, 2016, United States Senate, Bernie Sanders: U.S. Senator for Vermont. https://www.sanders.senate .gov/wp-content/uploads/sanders-cummings-letter-to-doj-ftc-on-insulin.pdf

"A recent review of off-label prescribing among office-based physicians found that 73 percent of off-label prescribing had little or no scientific support": R. S. Stafford, "Regulating Off-Label Drug Use—Rethinking the Role of the FDA." *New England Journal of Medicine* 358, no. 14, April 3, 2008.

"Currently, the reporting of adverse events is not mandated, but done on a voluntary basis, leading to vast underreporting": P. C. Hébert, D. Fergusson, and M. B. Stanbrook, "Off-Label Use of Recombinant Factor VIIa: Why We Need Better Drug Monitoring." *Canadian Medical Association Journal* 183, vol. 1, Jan. 11, 2011. https://doi.org/10.1503/cmaj.101842

POSTSCRIPT: THE LEFT SIDE OF THE MENU

"Z-Medica was sold to Teleflex, a large medical device company based in Pennsylvania, for $500 million": Maria Rachal, "Teleflex Lines Up $525M to Buy Hemostat Specialist Z-Medica." *MedTech Dive*, Oct. 29, 2020. https://www.medtechdive.com/news/teleflex-lines-up-525m-to-buy-hemostat-specialist-z-medica/588006/

" 'When the [HemCon] patent died, each of you Board Members should have signed the letter and made personal calls to shareholders' ": Oregon Business Team, "Lawyer Blasts Bankrupt HemCon." *Oregon Business*, August 2, 2012. https://www.oregonbusiness.com/article/item/7828-lawyer-blasts-bankrupt-hemcon; Nigel Jaquiss, "The Scarlet Letter." *Willamette Week*, July 31, 2012. https://www.wweek.com/portland/article-19504-the-scarlet-letter.html

"Pop star Taylor Swift made international news when she said in 2019, 'I carry QuikClot army grade bandage dressing' ": "Taylor Swift 'Carries Stab Bandages' after Stalker Scares." BBC News, March 6, 2019. https://www.bbc.co.uk/news/entertainment-arts-47472507

"Before the Las Vegas shootings, every vehicle of that city's metropolitan police department was issued a trauma kit including Combat Gauze": *1 October After-Action Review* (Las Vegas: Las Vegas Metropolitan Police Department, 2019). https://www.lvmpd.com/en-us/Documents/1_October_AAR_Final_0606 2019.pdf

"Sergeant Kennedy noted that Detective William Ghilarducci 'applied quick clot [sic]' ": Officer L. De Souza, Las Vegas Metropolitan Police Department Officer's Report, "Mandalay Bay Active Shooter," Oct. 6, 2017. https://archive.org/details/LVMPDOfficerReports

"Frank's consortium, now a mini empire, has been written up enthusiastically by the *Boston Globe* and *Condé Nast Traveler*": Christopher Muther, "How a Small Cape Cod Hotel Evolved into a $20 Million Resort." *Boston Globe*, March 17, 2022.

"The officer, Gerald Veneziano, still wearing street clothes, was driving a silver Volkswagen Passat": Alexi Friedman, "Fairfield Police Officer Recounts Night He Was Shot 6 Times." *Star-Ledger*, Oct. 21, 2010; "Manhunt for Suspects in Shooting of Officer in New Jersey." *New York Times*, Jan. 31, 2010.

Index

acidosis, 20
Aerodrome, 129–30
Aesop, 53–54
   Afghanistan War
   blood clotting trial for Marine Corps
      and, 52
   component therapy and, 211–12
   Factor Seven use and, 158, 161, 207
   fibrin bandages and, 25
   John Holcomb and, xx, 145, 209
   QuikClot use and, 127–28, 172
   whole blood transfusions and, 212
Aidid, Mohamed, xi–xiv
AK-47 rifles, 131
Alam, Hasan
   blood clotting trial for Marine Corps
      and, 44–46, 51, 52, 54, 64, 71,
      72, 85, 86, 229
   on Factor Seven, 157, 158–59, 187
   hemorrhagic shock research of, 51–
      52
   on QuikClot, 71, 87, 123, 135
   on zeolite, 45, 46, 52, 53, 62, 124
Aledort, Louis, 160
American Civil War, 14, 194
American Red Cross, 21–22, 25, 26, 81,
      145, 210
American Revolution, 83
anesthesia, advances in, 14

Aquinas, Thomas, 75, 77
AR-15 rifles, 129, 130–31
ArmaLite Corporation, 130
Artificial Organs, 160
Aykroyd, Dan, 131

Babe (film), 225
Baltimore Sun, 143, 165, 167, 169–70,
      171, 185–87
bedsores, 234–35
Belushi, John, 131
Benoit, David, 135
Bible, on blood, 15
Bick, Rodger, 158–60
bin Laden, Osama, xviii
Black, Ian, 190–97, 198, 207–8, 213,
      214
Black Hawk Down (film), 24–25, 40
Blajchman, Morris, 155–56
Blascom, Steven, 119–20, 172–73, 200–
      201
blood. *See also* traumatic bleeding
   clotting cascade, 19, 107, 137, 146,
      158
   clotting processes of, 7–8, 19–21,
      149–52, 158–59
   clotting proteins, 7, 8, 12, 17, 19–21,
      23, 107, 158
   component therapy and, 211

blood (*cont.*)
    cultural understanding of, 15
    fibrin clot of, 17, 19, 20
    kaolin's blood clotting properties,
        201–2
    properties of, 15, 19–20
    tranexamic acid and, 213
    whole blood transfusion and, 210–12
    zeolite's blood clotting properties, 7–
        10, 12, 31, 33–34, 37, 45, 46, 51,
        53, 63–64, *63*, 107, 109, 137,
        202, 235
blood clotting products
    development of, 18, 19, 21, 22–26,
        26, 40–42, 145–52
    for hemophilia patients, 148, 149
    thromboembolic events and, 155
blood transfusions, 14, 210–12
Bordas, Jean, 197
Boston Marathon bombing, 229
Bowden, Mark, xvii, 23–24
British army, Factor Seven and, 160,
    163, 187
British Medical Journal, 160
Brooke Army Medical Center, San
    Antonio, 190–91
Bureau of Medicine and Surgery, 110
Burkhard, Thomas, 110, 112
Bush, George W., 110, 112

cancer treatments, advances in,
    14–15
Carnegie, Dale, 174
Carter, James, 76
Catholic Charities, 36
Catto, William, 123
Center for Translational Injury Re-
    search, 189
chemotherapy, advances in, 14–15
chitosan, 26, 86, 229
Clinton, Bill, xviii
coagulopathy (impaired clot formation),
    20

Coakley, Timothy
    battlefield medicine conferences and,
        103–7, 109, 111, 114, 126
    court-martial investigation against,
        110–13
    Joseph Dacorta and, 103–4, 106–8,
        220
    education of, 94–96
    father of, 94–95
    in Iraq War, 89–94, 96–103, 112,
        113, 218
    marriage and family of, 96, 97, 101,
        103, 109, 218
    Naval service of, 95, 96–102, 218–19
    post-traumatic stress disorder and, 218
    QuikClot and, 90–91, 94, 101–9,
        110, 218
    QuikClot Combat Gauze and, 219
    QuikClot promotion and, 134
    QuikClot research proposals and, 94,
        108, 109, 110, 111, 137
    QuikClot trainings and, 109–10, 126
    Recovering Warrior Task Force and,
        219
    savant syndrome and, 109
    skepticism of, 90
    as surgeon for Navy Expeditionary
        Combat Command, 218–19
    as target of US Army, 104–6, 113
    traumatic brain injuries and, 108–9,
        218
Collaborating Centre on Research and
    Training in Injury Control, World
    Health Organization, 160
Columbia University, 162
Combat Casualty Care Research
    Program, Fort Detrick, Maryland,
    154
Combat Hospital (documentary), 143
Committee on Tactical Combat Casu-
    alty Care, 121, 205
Constant, Gus, 61
Cowen, Michael, 22

Dacorta, Joseph
    battlefield medicine conferences and,
        81–82, 103–4, 106–7, 109
    Ian Black and, 191
    blood clotting trial for Marine Corps
        and, 43–44, 52, 64, 72–73, 85–87
    Timothy Coakley and, 103–4, 106–
        8, 220
    education of, 75, 77–78, 79
    Factor Seven and, 157, 158
    family background of, 73
    father of, 73–75
    FDA approval of zeolite and, 52, 64,
        70
    on fibrin bandages, 23
    Forward Resuscitative Surgical
        System (FRSS) and, 84–85, 116
    Michael Given and, 80–81
    Bart Gullong and, 226
    John Holcomb and, 81–82
    mother of, 73
    Navy career of, 72–73, 76–84, 97,
        220
    patents of, 220
    in Peace Corps, 75–76
    on QuikClot, 135, 137, 138, 219
    QuikClot product development and,
        65, 67, 70, 71, 87–88, 108, 128
    retirement of, 219–20
    skepticism of, 73–76, 78, 81, 88
    Galen Stucky's kaolin studies and,
        203
Darwin, Charles, 79
Demetriades, Demetrios, 16, 187–88
Descartes, René, 78
DNA technology, 150
Doonesbury (comic strip), 136
Dorlac, Warren, 159
Drohan, William, 22
Durbin, Dick, 186
Dutton, Richard, 152
DW Healthcare Partners, 223–24
Dzik, Walter, 159

Eagles, Thomas
    blood clotting trial for Marine Corps
        and, 64–65, 72
    Timothy Coakley and, 107, 110, 220
    death of, 220
    family background of, 39
    FDA approval of QuikClot and, 70
    Bart Gullong and, 38–41, 43, 64, 65,
        221
    individual first-aid kit (IFAK)
        redesign, 84
    Marine Corps service of, 38–40, 80,
        81–83
    POGS machine and, 38
    QuikClot and, 65, 67, 71, 220–21
    Vietnam War and, 39, 64, 220
Egypt, 76
Emergency Ward Surgery, xx
Emerson, Fred, 59–60

Factor Seven (Recombinant Factor
    VIIa)
    adverse events in off-label injections,
        162, 212, 215
    Afghanistan War and, 158, 161, 207
    Hasan Alam on, 157, 158–59, 187
    Rodger Bick on, 159–60
    Ian Black on, 191, 192–93
    Boffard study of, 154–56
    clinical trials on, 162, 187, 188
    complications in use with soldiers,
        159–60, 161, 187, 192
    conceptual problem concerning,
        158–59
    fall of, 152, 187–88
    FDA on, 154, 156, 162, 163, 186–
        87, 192, 197, 214, 215
    Ulla Hedner's development of, 147–
        52, 164, 214
    John Holcomb on, 141, 145, 146–47,
        152, 154, 156–57, 160–61, 163–
        64, 170, 186–87, 192, 210,
        216–17

Factor Seven (*cont.*)
IED wounds and, 159, 161
Iraq War and, 157, 158, 161, 163–
67, 192, 195, 207
lack of studies on, 192
legacy of, 212
Robert Little on, 170
Caleb Lufkin and, 145–47, 162, 164
–65, 169, 212
Uri Martinowitz's case study on, 152
–54
Barbara Mikulski on, 185
Ian Roberts on, 153–54
sales of, 164
traumatic bleeding and, 152–55,
187, 212
US Army and, 156, 157, 158, 160,
161, 163–64, 170, 190, 193, 195,
205
whistleblower lawsuits against, 190–
91, 193–97, 207–8, 213–14
Factor Eight, 149
Factor Nine, 149
Factor Ten, 149
False Claims Act, 193–95
Fareed, Jawed, 158
Fast Act Bovine Clotting factor, 85
FDA (Food and Drug Administration)
adverse event reporting and, 215
on Factor Seven, 154, 156, 162, 163,
186–87, 192, 197, 214, 215
fibrin bandages approval and, 22, 23
HemCon approval and, 71
Parke-Davis and, 194
QuikClot approval and, 70, 137
restrictions on medical technologies,
xix
on Victoza, 214–15
zeolite approval and, 52–53, 64, 70
Feres doctrine, 169
fibrin bandages
failure of, 81, 145, 210
grants for, 235

John Holcomb and, xix, 19, 21,
22–26, 81, 156, 210
fibrin glue, 21–22
fibrinogen, 21
fibrin powder, 21–22
fibrin sheet foam, 21–22
Fishbein, Morris, 73–74
fluid resuscitation, 52
Forty-Sixth Combat Support Hospital,
xiv–xv, xvi, 13, 14, 24–25
Forward Resuscitative Surgical Systems
(FRSS), 37, 84–85, 116
Francis X. and Nancy Hursey Center
for Advanced Engineering and
Health Professions, 233–34
Franklin, David, 194

Garmatz, Edward A., 190
Gawande, Atul, 159
Ghilarducci, William, 229–30
Giffords, Gabby, 209
Given, Michael
Hasan Alam and, 52
Timothy Coakley and, 107–8
Joseph Dacorta and, 80–81
Factor Seven and, 157, 162–63
on QuikClot Combat Gauze, 206
Galen Stucky's kaolin studies and,
203
Vietnam War and, 42
Goethe, Johann Wolfgang von, 15
Gorsline, Marcy, 168–70
Gregory, Kenton, 26
Gulf War, 78–79, 84, 97
Gullong, Bart
antidepressants taken by, 175
battlefield medicine conferences and,
109, 114, 126–27, 129, 133, 172
Steven Blascom and, 119–20, 172–
73, 200–201
blood clotting trial for Marine Corps
and, 40–47, 51, 52, 62–65, *63*,
66, 86–87

boats of, 115

breakdown of, 171–80, 198, 200, 227

Timothy Coakley and, 104, 110, 114

criticism as "war profiteer," 172

Joseph Dacorta and, 226

Thomas Eagles and, 38–41, 43, 64, 65, 221

early career of, 29–30

early life of, 55–56, 73

education of, 28, 53, 55–59, 222

as entrepreneur, 29, 62, 116, 175, 180, 226

Factor Seven and, 158, 171–72

father's relationship with, 34, 57, 58, 59, 180–81, 182, 226–27

Florida and, 178–79, 198–200, 201, 226

John Holcomb and, 140–41, 142, 179, 180, 182, 189, 198

Frank Hursey and, 28, 30, 31–36, 40, 54, 114, 116–19, 135, 147, 174–75, 176, 177–78, 180, 198, 200–201, 205, 206–7, 223–25, 226, 228, 230–31, 232, 235–36

Iraq War consulting contract and, 175–77, 179–82

on Caleb Lufkin, 171, 182

marriage of, 29, 33, 35, 40, 47, 114–16, 171, 172–73, 175, 176, 178–79, 199, 200, 205

mother's relationship with, 34, 55, 57

On-Site Gas Systems responsibilities of, 34–39, 173–74, 180, 198

patent on nitrogen lowering oxygen level in liquid and, 117–18

Pentagon proposal for portable surgical centers and, 37–38

perceptions of people, 51, 118–19

philanthropy of, 228

POGS machine and, 38–39, 40, 45, 84–85, 116–17, 126, 173

post-traumatic stress disorder of, 181–82, 230

QuikClot as zeolite product name and, 65–66

QuikClot Combat Gauze and, 204–5, 206, 222, 230

QuikClot marketing and, 132–39, 179

QuikClot product booths and, 104, 109, 121, 126, 133, 172

QuikClot product design and production, 66–68, 71, 128–29, 131–32, 198–99

retirement of, 226–28

as rower and rowing coach, 28–29, 38, 46, 54, 55–57, 59–62, 180, 182, 238

as salesman, 29, 30–31, 34, 35–36, 46–48, 58, 60, 65, 115, 116–17, 119, 132, 173, 180

self-image of, 53–55, 114–15, 179–81, 182, 199, 230–31

speedometer for rowing shells and, 29, 46–47

on zeolite, 31, 33, 40, 52–53, 62–63, 132, 137

zeolite patent and, 68–71

zeolite studies and, 124–25

Z-Medica responsibilities of, 116, 119–21, 126, 127, 172–73, 175, 176, 178, 198, 200–201, 205

Z-Medica sale and, 223–25

Gullong, Linda

  in Florida, 175, 178–79

  Bart Gullong's marriage to, 29, 33, 35, 40, 47, 114–16, 171, 172–73, 175, 176, 178–79, 199, 200, 205, 227

Gullong, Sarah

  in Florida, 175, 198

  Bart Gullong's relationship as father and, 36, 47, 114–15, 132, 173, 198, 221, 222, 227, 231

Halloran General Hospital, Staten Island, New York, 17–18

Harder, Bob, 129

Hargrove, Dan, 193–94

heart attacks, blood clots causing, 21

Hedner, Ulla, Factor Seven developed by, 147–52, 164, 214

HemCon
 bankruptcy of, 27, 228–29
 battlefield medicine conferences and, 81–82, 103–7
 blood clotting trial for Marine Corps and, 85–86
 development of, 26, 27, 28, 122, 145, 235
 effectiveness of, 70, 82, 85, 86, 122–23, 188
 FDA approval of, 71
 John Holcomb and, 26, 81–82, 141, 156, 157, 188, 210
 suits against, 229
 US Army and, 26–27, 70–71, 81–82, 104, 105, 106, 121–22, 127, 141, 156, 157, 158, 170, 188, 204–5

hemophilia, 146, 148–50, 156, 162, 164, 187, 214

hemorrhage control. *See also* traumatic bleeding
 Hasan Alam's research on hemorrhagic shock, 51–52
 John Holcomb on, xix
 uncontrolled hemorrhage as cause of death, 17

hemostatic agents
 blood clotting trial for Marine Corps and, 52, 85–86
 FDA approval of QuikClot and, 70
 HemCon and, 121–22
 for hemophilia patients, 146, 148–50
 as medical devices, 145
 traumatic bleeding and, 26, 41
 zeolite as, 41–42

hepatitis, transmission of, 19, 22

Hepburn, Katharine, 34

HIV, 150, 212

Holcomb, John
 battlefield medicine conferences and, 126–27
 on Battle of Mogadishu, xviii, 14, 210–11
 Ian Black's whistleblower lawsuit against Novo Nordisk and, 190, 195
 at Center for Translational Injury Research, 189
 combat experience of, 14
 as commander at Institute of Surgical Research, 18–19, 145, 156, 188–89, 192, 195, 205, 209, 210
 on component therapy, 211
 Defense Subcommittee testimony of, 170, 186
 as director of army trauma medicine, xx, 107
 early life of, xv, 14
 education of, xv–xvi, 14
 on Factor Seven, 141, 145, 146–47, 152, 154, 156–57, 158, 160–61, 163–64, 170, 186–87, 192, 210, 216–17
 fibrin bandage developed by, xix, 19, 21, 22–26, 156, 210
 Bart Gullong and, 140–41, 142, 179, 180, 182, 189, 198
 Ulla Hedner compared to, 148–49
 HemCon bandages and, 26, 81–82, 141, 156, 157, 188, 210
 Iraq War and, xx, 145, 157, 209
 on leadership philosophy, 19
 legacy of, 209–10
 Robert Little and, 165
 Mogadishu casualties and, xiv–xvii, xx, 13, 14, 24–25, 127, 147, 148
 persuasive speaking abilities of, 13–14
 on PolyHeme, 210

on QuikClot, 70, 126–27, 140–41, 158
on QuikClot Combat Gauze, 205, 207
resignation from Institute of Surgical Research, 189, 207
on tourniquets, 165, 209, 210
trauma research of, xviii–xx, 15, 16–19, 26–27, 51, 81–82
at University of Texas medical school, 189, 208–9
on zeolite, 124
Hufstader, Robert, 71
Hursey, Frank
blood clotting trial for Marine Corps and, 40–42, 44, 45, 46, 63–64, 63, 65, 87
Bosnian refugees hired by, 36
businesses of, 5, 8, 10–12, 28, 30, 31–35, 114, 116–19
Timothy Coakley and, 110
criticism as "war profiteer," 172
donation of medical oxygen generators to NYC firefighters, 36–37
education of, 3, 4, 5, 6, 233, 234
equanimity of, 174
Factor Seven and, 158, 171–72, 235
family background of, 3–5, 34
Bart Gullong and, 28, 30, 31–36, 40, 54, 114, 116–19, 135, 147, 174–75, 176, 177–78, 180, 198, 200–201, 205, 206–7, 223–25, 226, 228, 230–31, 232, 235–36
John Holcomb and, 189
inventions of, 8–9, 11, 12, 31, 119, 130, 136, 224
on kaolin, 201–4, 235
limousine company of, 232
marriage and family life of, 3, 4, 5, 7–9, 11–12, 42–43
as mechanical engineer, 3, 4, 5–6, 12, 32, 116
patent on nitrogen lowering oxygen

level in liquid and, 117–18
philanthropy of, 231, 233–34
POGS machine and, 38, 84, 116–17, 235
pressure swing technology and, 6, 35, 235
QuikClot as zeolite product name and, 65–66
QuikClot Combat Gauze and, 204–5, 222, 230
QuikClot product design and production and, 66–68, 71, 128, 235
real estate investments of, 232–33
work life of, 173
on zeolite, 6–12, 31, 33–34, 37, 40, 44, 46, 53, 65, 68, 109, 137, 202–3, 231, 234–35
zeolite patent and, 10, 12, 68–71
Hursey, Nancy, 3–5, 7–9, 11–12, 42, 173, 231–34
Hursey Resort in Soroti, 231–32
Hussein, Saddam, 99, 142
hypothermia, 20

IEDs (improvised explosive devices), 93–94, 100, 139, 159, 161
Institute of Surgical Research (ISR), San Antonio, Texas
Ian Black as researcher at, 190, 192
care of combat casualties and, 17–18
Factor Seven and, 156, 195, 216–17
fibrin bandage and, 21, 23–24
Bart Gullong and, 116
HemCon and, 26
John Holcomb as commander of, 18–19, 145, 156, 188–89, 192, 195, 205, 209, 210
John Holcomb as researcher at, 17, 18
Shawn Nessen as commander of, 19
Office of Naval Research compared to, 80

Institute of Surgical Research (*cont.*)
  on QuikClot, 105, 121
  on QuikClot Combat Gauze, 206
  zeolite study of, 124, 125
insulin, 150, 157, 215
interservice rivalries, 70, 82–84, 97
Iraq War
  battlefield medicine innovations and, 109
  Ian Black and, 191–92
  Bush/Kerry election as referendum on, 110, 112–13
  Timothy Coakley in, 89–94, 96–103, 112, 113, 218
  component therapy and, 211–12
  Factor Seven use and, 157, 158, 161, 163–67, 192, 195, 207
  Forward Resuscitative Surgical Systems (FRSS) and, 85
  Bart Gullong's consulting contract in, 175–77, 179–82
  John Holcomb and, xx, 145, 157, 209
  Caleb Lufkin's injuries and, 142–44, 166
  medical experiments on injured soldiers in, 195
  QuikClot Combat Gauze use and, 206
  QuikClot use and, 87–88, 121, 125, 126, 127–28, 135–36, 138–40, 176, 199
  Tenth Combat Support Hospital and, 142–44
  US Marines and, 83–84, 135
Israel Defense Force, Medical Corps, 203–4
Israeli army, 147, 152, 157, 162–63, 187–88

JAMA: The Journal of the American Medical Association, 25, 162, 163
Johnson, Louis, 83

Joint Commission on Accreditation of Healthcare Organizations (JCAHO), xix
Journal of Trauma, 18, 124, 155–56, 163, 209

kaolin, Frank Hursey on, 201–4, 235
kaolin clotting test (KCT), 202
Kennedy, John F., 131
Kerry, John, 110, 112
Krause, David, 70
Kules, Ryan, 138–40

Lancet, 153–54, 160
Landstuhl Regional Medical Center, Germany, 159, 165, 167
Langley, Samuel, 129–30
Larson, Gary, 118
Leave no man behind maxim, xiii–xiv
Legan, Joe, 124
Levinson, Jay Conrad, 132
Lincoln, Abraham, 194
Lincoln Law, 193–94
Little, Robert, 143, 165, 167, 169–70, 171, 185–87
Lufkin, Caleb
  death of, 147, 169, 171, 185
  early life of, 143
  Factor Seven and, 145–47, 162, 164–65, 169, 212
  funeral of, 167–70
  Bart Gullong on, 171, 182
  Iraq War injuries of, 142–44, 166
  at Landstuhl Regional Medical Center, 165, 167–68
  surgery and treatment of, 165
  at Tenth Combat Support Hospital, 142, 143–45, 165
  at Walter Reed hospital, 167–69
Lufkin, Tammy, 169

M-16 rifles, 129, 130–31
McKinley, William, 129
McNamara, Robert, 131

Mahaffee, Shane, 165–67, 170, 171, 185, 212

Mahaffee, Skip, 167

Maiman, Earle, 58

Mandalay Bay hotel shootings, Las Vegas, 229–30

Marine Corps Warfighting Laboratory, Quantico, Virginia, xix, 38, 79–81, 82

Marine Polymer Technologies, 86, 229

Martinowitz, Uri, 147–48, 152–54

Massachusetts General Hospital, Boston, 187

Mayer, Stephan, 159

Mayo, William, 14

Med-Equip, 43, 66, 86

medical science liaisons, 193, 194

Memorial Hermann-Texas Medical Center, 209

Mikulski, Barbara, 185–87

Mogadishu, Battle of, xi–xviii, xx, 13, 14, 15, 24, 76, 210–11

Monro Mufflers, 35

Montiel, Oscar, 193–95, 197, 198, 207–8, 214

Mount Sinai Hospital, 160

Nakamura, Terri, 196–97

National Institute of Allergy and Infectious Diseases, 17

National Institutes of Health, 52, 108

natural selection, 79

Naval Medical Research Center, 124

Navy Surgeon General, 108

Navy Trauma Training Center, 122

Nessen, Shawn, 19

Neurontin, 194

New England Journal of Medicine, 154, 159, 162, 163, 186–87

New York Times, 135, 160–61, 163, 213

9/11, 2001 attacks, 36–37, 51, 97

Nordisk Insulinlaboratorium, 150

North American Rescue, 104

North American Treaty Organization (NATO), xi–xii, 76

NovoLog, 215

Novo Nordisk
  clinical trial of Factor Seven, 154–56
  Columbia University randomized clinical trial funded by, 162
  Factor Seven produced by, 145, 150–51, 157, 164, 213, 214, 215
  Ulla Hedner as research scientist for, 150
  insulin manufactured by, 150, 157, 215
  marketing of, 154, 156, 193, 214–15
  Orphan Drug Act and, 151
  US Army and, 156–57, 193, 216–17
  Victoza and, 214–15
  whistleblower lawsuits against, 190–91, 193–97, 207–8, 213–14

Office of Naval Research (ONR)
  blood clotting trial for Marine Corps and, 42, 52
  Joseph Dacorta and, 79–80, 86, 157
  QuikClot research and, 108, 137
  Galen Stucky's kaolin studies and, 203

Office of the Secretary of Defense, xix

Olson, Eric, 189

On-Site Gas Systems
  Bart Gullong considered for, 28, 30–33
  Bart Gullong's responsibilities at, 34–39, 173–74, 180, 198
  Frank Hursey and, 10–11, 231
  POGS machine and, 38, 40, 84, 116–17, 118, 119, 126, 173, 235
  profits of, 53

Operation Deny Flight, 76

Oregon Medical Laser Center, 26

Orphan Drug Act, 151

Pace, Peter, 64–65, 221

Parke-Davis, 194

Parkland school shooting, Florida, 229
Patton, George, 74, 138
Peake, James, 209
Peale, Norman Vincent, 4
Pelham House Resort, 232
Pentagon
    Dick Durbin and, 186
    9/11 attacks and, 51
    proposal request for portable surgical
        centers, 37
    trauma research funding and, xx
Persian Gulf War, xvii–xviii
Phan, Sanh, 10–12, 32, 37–38, 116,
    119
POGS (Portable Oxygen Generating
    System), 38, 40, 84, 116–19, 126,
    173, 235
PolyHeme, 210
Popper, Karl, 79, 81, 85
pressure swing technology, 6, 35, 235
Pruitt, Basil, 18, 209
pulmonary embolisms, 21
Pusateri, Anthony, 26

QuikClot
    Timothy Coakley and, 90–91, 94,
        101–9, 110, 218
    heat produced by, 105, 109, 123–28,
        201, 203
    HemCon compared to, 71, 123
    Iraq War use and, 87–88, 121, 125,
        126, 127–28, 135–36, 138–40,
        176, 199
    kaolin formulation used for, 201–4
    marketing of, 132–39
    product design and development, 65,
        66–68, 70, 71, 87–88, 107, 145,
        198–99
    product promotion and, 121, 133–37
    silver-enhanced versions of, 137,
        203
    testing against safety standards,
        67–68

US Army on, 116, 121, 126, 127,
    128–29, 132–34, 138, 170, 171,
    173, 179, 220
as zeolite product name, 65–66
Z-Medica's manufacturing of, 70,
    119–20, 137
QuikClot Combat Gauze, 204–5, 206,
    219, 222, 229–30

R. Adams Cowley Shock Trauma
    Center, Baltimore, 162–63
RAND Corporation, xix, 16, 163,
    187
Rapid Deployment Hemostat Bandage,
    85–86
Reagan, Ronald, 95
Recombinant Factor VIIa (Factor
    Seven). *See* Factor Seven (Recombi-
    nant Factor VIIa)
Recovering Warrior Task Force, 219
Rhee, Peter, 122, 125
Roberts, Ian, 153–54, 160, 212–13
Roberts, Preye, 236
Royal Centre for Defence Medicine,
    163
RPGs (rocket-propelled grenades), xiii,
    xiv
Rwanda, xviii, 76, 78

San Antonio Express-News, 196–97
Sancredi, Rachel, 133–35, 137–38
Sanofi, 215
Scientific American, 136, 235
scientific method, 79
Secrease, Seth, 128
Shakespeare, William, 15, 53
Shooter (film), 136–37
Shorr, Andrew, 161
shrimp shells, hemostatic properties of,
    26, 71
Siegel, Jamie, 214
Smith, Jamie, 24–25, 40, 43, 236,
    237–38

Somalia, Battle of Mogadishu, xi–xviii, xx, 13, 14, 15, 24, 76, 210–11
Stahancyk, Jody, 229
Steinbruner, David, 144
Stewart, Jimmy, 106
Stoner, Eugene, 130–31
strokes, blood clots causing, 21
Stucky, Galen, 137, 203–4, 206
Swift, Taylor, 229
syphilis, 212

Tenth Combat Support Hospital, 142, 143–45, 165, 166, 187
thrombin, 21
thromboembolic events, 155
tissue factor, in blood clotting process, 149
tourniquets
   John Holcomb's advocacy for, 165, 209, 210
   medics' use in field, 128, 139, 143, 145
   QuikClot Combat Gauze and, 22, 205
tranexamic acid, 213
TraumaDex, 85
traumatic bleeding
   biochemical methods of speeding up clotting process, 17
   evidence-based practices for, 212–13
   experimental treatments for, 16
   Factor Seven and, 152–55, 187, 212
   hemostatic agents and, 26, 41
   John Holcomb's research on, xviii–xx, 15, 16–19, 26–27, 51, 81–82
   informed consent of patients and, 16
   Ian Roberts on, 153
   tools and techniques for stopping, xvii, xix, 13, 14, 15–17, 21–22, 26–27
   uncontrolled hemorrhage as cause of death, 17
Trudeau, Garry, 136

T.R.U.E. Research Foundation for the Advancement of Military Medicine, 195–97, 207
Truman, Harry, 83
Twenty-Eighth Combat Support Hospital, Baghdad, 191

Ukraine, 76, 219
Uniformed Services University of the Health Sciences, 123
US Air Force
   AR-15 rifle and, 131
   on HemCon, 123
   portable surgical centers proposal of, 37–38
   QuikClot and, 124
   on zeolite, 124–25
US Army. *See also* Institute of Surgical Research (ISR), San Antonio, Texas
   Army Rangers at Mogadishu, xi–xvii, xx, 24–25
   Timothy Coakley targeted by, 104–6, 113
   Factor Seven and, 156, 157, 158, 160, 161, 163–64, 170, 190, 193, 195, 205
   fibrin bandages used by, 22–23, 156
   HemCon bandages and, 26–27, 70–71, 81–82, 104, 105, 106, 121–22, 127, 141, 156, 157, 158, 170, 188, 204–5
   hemostasis program of, 26
   M-16 rifle favored by, 130–31
   Medical Command of, 17
   Medical Research and Materiel Command, Fort Detrick, 116
   medical supplies of, 97
   military insiders as contractors and, 129–30
   Novo Nordisk and, 156–57, 193, 216–17
   Ordnance Corps, 131
   personnel of, 84

US Army (*cont.*)
  POGS and, 116
  on QuikClot, 116, 121, 126, 127, 128–29, 132–34, 138, 170, 171, 173, 179, 220
  QuikClot Combat Gauze and, 204–5, 206
  zeolite study of, 124
US Army Medical Research Institute of Chemical Defense, Maryland, 17
US Army Research Institute of Environmental Medicine, Massachusetts, 17
US Army Training and Doctrine Command, xix
US Department of Defense, xix–xx, 78, 106, 129–30, 169, 206, 207, 219
US Department of Justice, 194, 196, 207, 213–15
US Marine Corps
  blood clotting trial for, 40–47, 51, 52, 54, 62–65, *63*, 71, 72, 85–86, 87, 229
  equipment and supplies for, 97
  on HemCon, 123
  Iraq War and, 83–84, 135
  mission of, 82–83
  QuikClot and, 157, 173
  US Army compared to, 83–84
US Navy
  Joseph Dacorta and, 72–73, 76–84, 97, 220
  QuikClot and, 157, 173
  QuikClot kaolin product and, 204
US Patent and Trademark Office, 10, 12, 68
US Special Operations Command, 189
United States v. Novo Nordisk, 190–97, 207–8
US War Department, 129–30
University of Padua, Italy, 160
University of Texas Medical School in Austin, 189
UN peacekeepers, xviii

Vandre, Robert, 154
Veneziano, Gerald, 236–38
Victoza, 214–15
Vietnam War
  Battle of Mogadishu compared to, xiv
  component therapy and, 211
  Thomas Eagles and, 39, 64, 220
  frozen blood products used in, 15
  Michael Given and, 42
  Bart Gullong and, 58, 176
  M-16 and AR-15 rifles debate and, 129, 130–31

Wahlberg, Mark, 136–37
Walter Reed hospital, 159, 167–68
Warfighter Performance Department, 42
Warner, John, 110
Washington, George, 83
Waters Kraus & Paul, 193–94
Watson, James, 74
Watson, Paul, xvii, xviii
Wayne, John, 127
Webert, Kathryn, 155–56
Whitman, Walt, 75
Wilson, Gregory, 128
Wolfe, Sidney, 208
World War I, 14–15, 21–22
World War II, 14–15, 21–22, 74–75, 83
Wounded Warrior Project, 140
Wright, Orville, 129–30
Wright, Wilbur, 129–30

Yom Kippur War, 147

zeolite
  blood clotting properties of, 7–10, 12, 31, 33–34, 37, 45, 46, 51, 53, 63–64, *63*, 107, 109, 137, 202, 235
  heat generated by, 9–10, 87, 105, 109, 123, 124–25, 128, 137, 201

Frank Hursey's directions for use, 41–42

Frank Hursey's study of, 6–12, 31, 33–34, 37, 40, 44, 46, 53, 65, 68, 109, 137, 202–3, 231, 234–35

Frank Hursey's testing for safety, 37

industrial uses of, 6–7, 31, 53

as medical device, 64, 145

New York Times on, 135

Z-Medica

DW Healthcare Partners' purchase of, 223–25

Bart Gullong's responsibilities at,

116, 119–21, 126, 127, 172–73, 175, 176, 178, 198, 200–201, 205

hospital market and, 223, 228

naming of, 66

QuikClot Combat Gauze and, 204–6, 222, 223, 228, 238

QuikClot kaolin formation and, 201–4

QuikClot manufactured by, 70, 119–20, 137

Teleflex's purchase of, 228

US Army and, 220

About the Author

Charles Barber is a writer in residence at Wesleyan University, a lecturer in psychiatry at the Yale School of Medicine, and the author of the critically acclaimed books *Songs from the Black Chair, Comfortably Numb, Citizen Outlaw,* and *Peace & Health.* He was educated at Harvard and Columbia universities, and he lives in Connecticut with his family.

CharlesBarberWriting.com